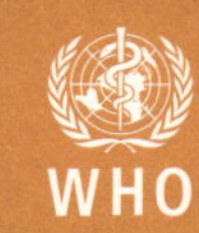

Women, Ageing and Health: A Framework for Action

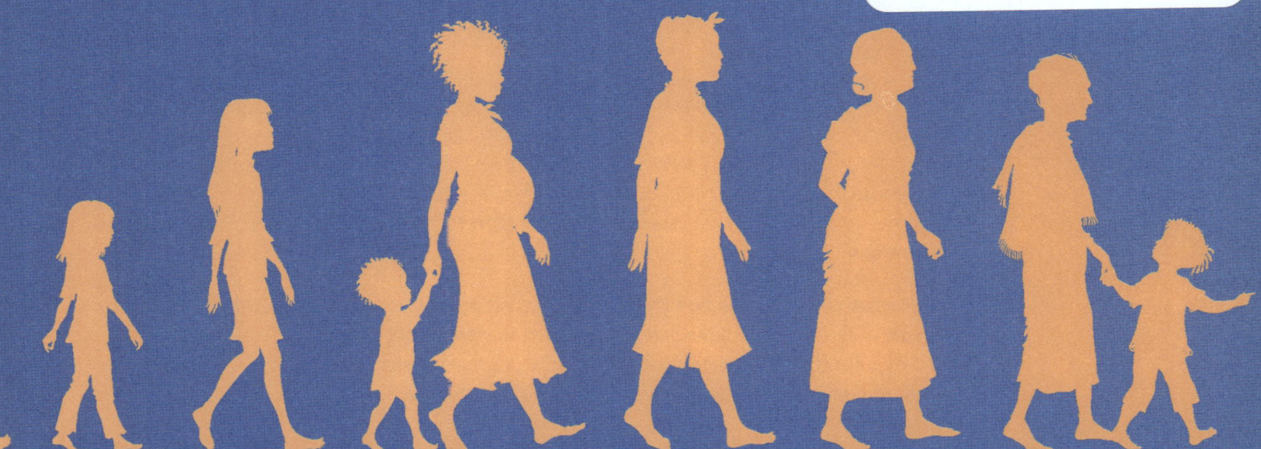

Focus on Gender

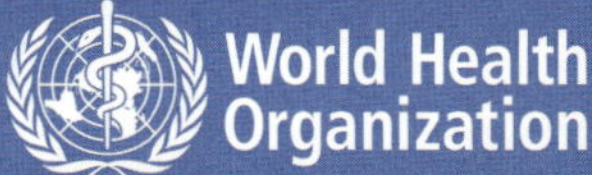

WHO Library Cataloguing-in-Publication Data

Women, ageing and health : a framework for action : focus on gender.

1.Ageing. 2.Women's health. 3.Longevity. 4.Women. 5.Gender identity. I.World Health Organization. II.United Nations Population Fund.

ISBN 978 92 4 156352 9   (NLM classification: WA 309)

Design: Langfeldesigns.com Marilyn Langfeld/Art Director, Adina Murch/Design, © Ann Feild/Didyk Illustration

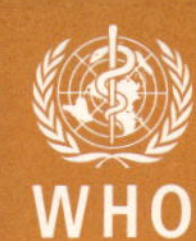

Contents

Acknowledgements

This report summarizes the evidence about women, ageing and health from a gender perspective and provides a framework for developing action plans to improve the health and well-being of ageing women.

This publication was developed by the Department of Ageing and Life Course (ALC) under the direction of Dr Alexandre Kalache and Irene Hoskins. ALC received support from Francois Farah and Ann Pawliczko from the Population and Development Branch of the United Nations Population Fund (UNFPA) and collaboration from Dr 'Peju Olukoya from the Department of Gender, Women and Health (GWH) of the World Health Organization (WHO).

The input and contribution of the following experts – who represented all WHO regions and provided background material – are gratefully acknowledged: Dr Isabella Aboderin (Nigeria), Prof. Nana Araba Apt (Ghana), Dr Narimah Awin (Malaysia), Dr Denise Eldemire-Shearer (Jamaica), Dr Randah R. Hamadeh (Bahrain) Dr Anita Liberalesso Neri (Brazil), Dr Indira Jai Prakash (India), Dr Mary Ann Tsao (Singapore), Dr Barbro Westerholm (Sweden) and Mahmoud Fathalla (Egypt). In addition, contribution from colleagues from international non-governmental organizations was gratefully received: Dr Jane Barratt (IFA), Dr Gloria Gutman (IAGG), Mark Gorman (HelpAge International)

The report was prepared based on a literature review available at: http://www.who.int/en/ageing/en compiled by Peggy Edwards, a health promotion consultant from Ottawa, Canada who, under the direction of the ALC Department, produced a draft of the report.

Taking action for older women and men

As they age, women and men share the basic needs and concerns related to the enjoyment of human rights such as shelter, food, access to health services, dignity, independence and freedom from abuse. The evidence shows however, that when judged in terms of the likelihood of being poor, vulnerable and lacking in access to affordable health care, older women merit special attention. While this publication focuses on the vulnerabilities and strengths of women at older ages, it is often difficult and sometimes undesirable to formulate recommendations that apply exclusively to women. Clearly many of the suggestions for action in this report apply to older men as well.

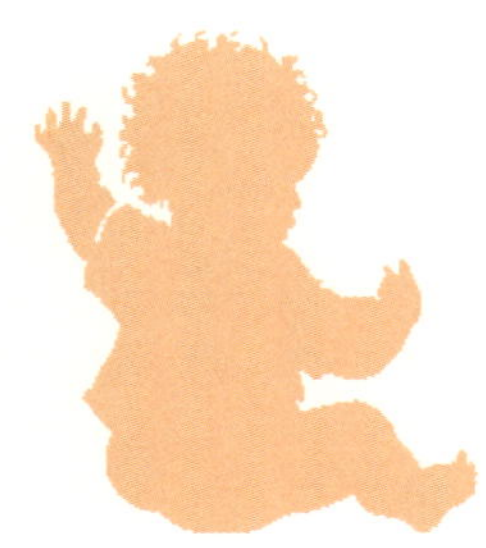

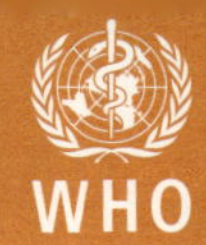

1. Introduction

> *"Gender is a 'lens' through which to consider the appropriateness of various policy options and how they will affect the well-being of both women and men."*
> … Active Ageing: A Policy Framework[1]
> World Health Organization, 2002

This framework for action addresses the health status and factors that influence women's health at midlife and older ages with a focus on gender. It provides guidance on how policy-makers, practitioners, nongovernmental organizations and civil society can improve the health and well-being of ageing women by simultaneously applying both a gender and an ageing lens in their policies, programmes and practices, as well as in research. A full review of the evidence is available in a longer complementary document entitled Women, Ageing and Health: A Review. Focus on Gender. It will be available online shortly at http://www.who.int/ageing/publications/gender/en/index.html

About this report

The concepts and principles in this document build on WHO's active ageing policy framework, which calls on policy-makers, practitioners, nongovernmental organizations and civil society to optimize opportunities for health, participation and security in order to enhance quality of life for people as they age.[1] This requires a comprehensive approach that takes into account the gendered nature of the life course.

This report endeavors to provide information on ageing women in both developing and developed countries; however, data are often scant in many areas of the developing world. Some implications and directions for policy and practice based on the evidence and known best practices are included in this report. These are intended to stimulate discussion and lead to specific recommendations and action plans. The report provides an overall framework for taking action that is useful in all settings (Chapter 2). Specific responses in policy, practice and research is undoubtedly best left to policy-makers, experts and older people in individual countries and regions, since they best understand the political, economic and social context within which decisions must be made.

This publication and the complementary longer Review are designed to contribute to the global review of progress since the Fourth World Conference on Women (Beijing, 1995),[2] the Madrid International Plan of Action on Ageing (2002),[3] and the implementation of the Millennium Development Goals.[4] While some progress has been made as a result of these United Nations initiatives and new policy directions have been adopted at the country level, the rights and contributions of older women remain largely invisible in most settings. This lack of visibility is especially problematic for ageing women who face multiple sources of disadvantage, including those who are poor, divorced or widowed; immigrants and refugees; and members of ethnic minorities.

Key concepts and terms in this report

Sex and gender. **Sex** refers to biology whereas **gender** refers to the social and economic roles, responsibilities and opportunities that society and families assign to women and men. Both sex and gender influence health risks, health-seeking behaviour, and health outcomes for men and women, thus influencing their access to health care systems and the response of those systems.[5]

Older women refers to women age 50 and older. **Ageing women** refers to the same chronological group but emphasizes that ageing is a process that occurs at very different rates among various individuals and groups. Privileged women may remain free of the health concerns that often accompany ageing until well into their 70s and 80s. Others who endure a lifetime of poverty, malnutrition and heavy labour may be chronologically young but functionally "old" at age 40. Decision-makers need to consider the contextual differences in how the process of ageing is experienced in their specific environment, when designing gender-responsive policies and programmes for ageing women.

Ageing is also both a biological and social construct. Physiological changes such as a reduction in bone density and visual acuity are a normal part of the ageing process. At the same time, socioeconomic factors such as living arrangements, income and access to health care greatly affect how individuals and populations experience ageing.

Ageing may also constitute a **continuum of independence, dependence and interdependence** that ranges from older women who are essentially independent and coping well with daily life, to those who require some assistance in their day-to-day lives, to those who are dependent on others for support and care. These groups are heterogeneous, reflecting diverse values, health status, educational levels and socioeconomic status.

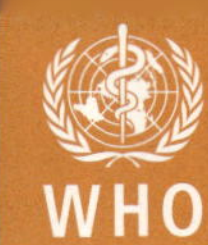

A global profile of ageing women

For multiple reasons the feminization of ageing has important policy implications for all countries:

- Ageing women make up a significant proportion of the world's population and their numbers are growing The number of women age 60 and over will increase from about 336 million in 2000 to just over 1 billion in 2050. Women outnumber men in older age groups and this imbalance increases with age. Worldwide, there are some 123 women for every 100 men aged 60 and over.[6]

- While the highest proportions of older women are in developed countries, the majority live in developing countries, where population ageing is occurring at a rapid pace.

- The fastest growing group among ageing women is the oldest-old (age 80-plus). Worldwide, by age 80 and over, there are 189 women for every 100 men. By age 100 and over, the gap reaches 385 women for every 100 men.[6] While most ageing women remain relatively healthy and independent until late in life, the very old most often require chronic care and help with day-to-day activities.

- Older women are a highly diverse group. Life at age 60 is obviously very different from life at age 85. Although cohorts of older women may experience some common situations, such as a shared political environment, exposure to war and the arrival of new technologies, their longevity has given them more time to develop unique biographies based on a lifetime of experiences.

> **Equity in health** means addressing the disparities between and among different groups of older women, as well as those between women and men.

The knowledge gap

When it comes to research and knowledge development, older women face double jeopardy — exclusion related to both sexism and ageism. Current information concerning ways in which gender and sex differences between women and men influence health in older age is inadequate. While gender-inclusive guidelines have been implemented in some countries, there is still a tendency for clinical studies to focus on men and exclude women. Surveillance data that include sex and age-disaggregated data are also limited. For example, most international studies on health issues – such as violence and HIV/AIDS – fail to compile statistics for people over the age of 50. Lastly, there is a paucity of research on gender differences in the social determinants of health. A recent study mapping existing research and knowledge gaps concerning the situation of older women in Europe found a lack of research related to women aged 50 to 60 in particular.[7] While there were numerous longitudinal studies on ageing, these studies had little or no gender analysis of the different impacts of health conditions and the social determinants of health on ageing women and men. In this report, some key issues for research and information of and are described in each chapter.

2. A framework for action

This chapter describes a gender- and age-responsive framework for action based on the following components:

- A life-course approach

- A determinants of health approach

- Three pillars for action

- A gender- and age-responsive lens

A life-course approach

Ageing is a lifelong process, which begins before we are born and continues throughout life. The functional capacity of our biological systems (e.g. muscular strength, cardiovascular performance, respiratory capacity) increases during the first years of life, reaches its peak in early adulthood and naturally declines thereafter. The slope of decline is largely determined by external factors throughout the life course. The natural decline in cardiac or respiratory function, for example, can be accelerated by factors such as smoking and air pollution, leaving an individual with lower functional capacity than would normally be expected at a particular age. Health in older age is therefore to the largest extent a reflection of the living circumstances and actions of an individual during the entire life span.[8]

This finding implies that individuals can influence how they age by practising healthier lifestyles and by adapting to age-associated changes. However, some life course factors may not be modifiable at the individual level. For instance, an individual may have little or no control over economic disadvantages and environmental threats that directly affect the ageing process and often predispose him or her to disease in later life.

Growing evidence supports the concept of critical periods of growth and development in utero and during early infancy and childhood when environmental insults may have lasting effects on disease risk in later life. For example, evidence suggests that poor growth in utero leads to a variety of chronic disorders such as cardiovascular disease, non-insulin dependent diabetes, and hypertension.[9] Exposures in later life may still influence disease risk in a simple additive way but it is argued that fetal exposures permanently alter anatomical structures and a variety of metabolic systems.[10] This means that girls who are born into societies that favour boys and deprive girls are particularly likely to experience disease and life.

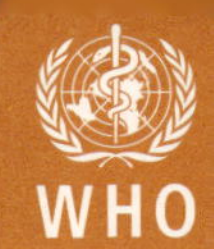

> **Examples of life course events that increase women's vulnerability to poor health in older age**
>
> - Gender discrimination against girls child leading to inequitable access to food and care by female and male infants and children.
>
> - Restrictions on education at all levels.
>
> - Childbirth without adequate health care and support.
>
> - Low incomes and inequitable access to decent work due to gender-discrimination in the labour force.
>
> - Caregiving responsibilities associated with mothering, grandmothering and looking after one's spouse and older parents that prevent or restrict working for an income and access to an employee-based pension.
>
> - Domestic violence, which may begin in childhood, continue in marriage and is a common form of elder abuse.
>
> - Widowhood, which commonly leads to a loss of income and may lead to social isolation.
>
> - Cultural traditions and attitudes that limit access to health care in older age, for example older women are much less likely than older men to receive cataract surgery in many countries.

A life-course perspective calls on policy-makers and civil society to invest in the various phases of life, especially at key transition points when risks to well-being and windows of opportunity are greatest. These include critical periods for both biological and social development, including in utero, the first six years of life, adolescence, transition from school to the workforce, motherhood, menopause, the onset of chronic illnesses and widowhood. Policies that reduce inequalities protect individuals at these critical times.[11]

Even with multiple changes in policies related to education and labour-market participation, gender-specified roles and careers interrupted because of childbearing and caregiving make it very difficult for women to earn as much as men in their respective lifetimes. Thus, the prevention and alleviation of poverty in older age calls for a set of policies based on a new paradigm that provides social safety nets at key times in the female life course, and particularly when women are unable to earn an adequate wage in the open labour market. This includes policies and practices that:

- support reproductive health and safe motherhood programmes;

- support girls' access to education with a special effort to enable their transition from primary to secondary and to post-secondary schooling;

- enable equitable entry to the labour market and to meaningful, protected work;

- provide incentives for 'family friendly' policies in the workplace which support pregnancy, breastfeeding, and caring for children and older family members;

- support caregivers of family members who are ill or frail, and ease the financial burden and employment opportunity costs of this essential role;

- support changes in work practice that enable older women to remain in both the formal and informal labour markets;

- support voluntary and gradual retirement as well as incentives to save for retirement and long-term care needs;

- ensure that equal rights to the inheritance of property and resources upon the death of a parent or spouse are upheld;

- ensure the right to health and equal access to health care;

- ensure that all older women have an income that satisfies the basic necessities of life, as well as equal access to required health, social, and legal services;

- provide additional support to widows as required, to older women who live alone, to those who are poor or disabled, and to those who require long-term care in or outside of the family residence; and

- support compassionate end-of-life care and help with arrangements for a peaceful death and appropriate burial required.

A determinants-of-health approach

There is now clear evidence that health care and biology are just two of the factors influencing health. The social, political, cultural, and physical conditions under which people live and grow older are equally important influences.[12]

Active ageing depends on a variety of "determinants" that surround individuals, families and nations. These factors directly or indirectly affect well-being, the onset and progression of disease and how people cope with illness and disability. The determinants of active ageing are interconnected in many ways and the interplay between them is important. For example, women who are poor (economic determinant) are more likely to be exposed to inadequate housing (physical determinant), societal violence (social determinant) and to not eat nutritious foods (behavioural determinant).

Figure 1 shows the major determinants of active ageing. Gender and culture are cross-cutting factors that affect all the others. For example, gender- and culture-related customs mean that men and women differ significantly when it comes to risk-taking and health-care-seeking behaviours. Culturally driven expectations affect how women experience menopause in various parts of the world. The gendered nature of caregiving and employment means that women are disadvantaged in the economic determinants of active ageing.

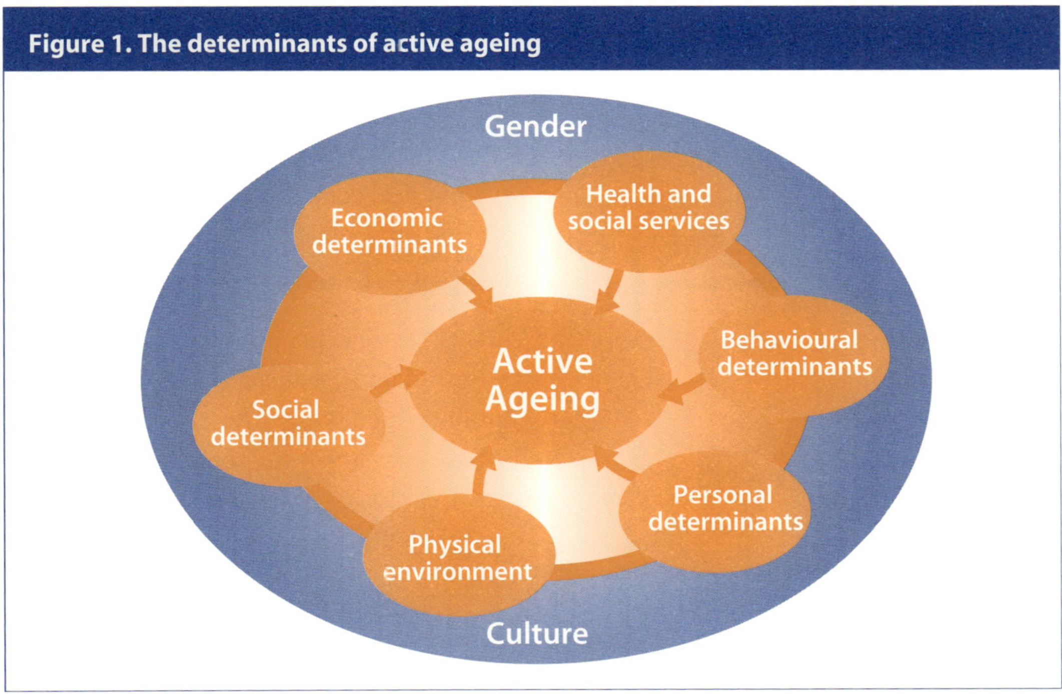

Source: *Active Ageing: A Policy Framework*, WHO, 2002 (http://www.who.int/ageing/publications/active/en/index.html)

Three pillars for action

The ideas presented in this report build on the WHO active ageing framework, which calls on policy-makers, service providers, nongovernmental organizations and civil society to take action in three areas or "pillars": participation, health and security (see Figure 2, next page). The policy framework for active ageing is guided by the United Nations Principles for Older People: independence, participation, care, self-fulfilment and dignity. Decisions are based upon an understanding of how the social, physical, personal and economic determinants of active ageing influence the way that individuals and populations age. This framework aims to reduce inequities in health by understanding the gendered nature of the life course.

The priority areas for action described in Chapter 10 of this report are grouped under the three pillars.

Active ageing is the process of optimizing opportunities for health, participation and security in order to enhance quality of life as people age.[1]

The gender- and age-responsive lens

Under the active ageing framework, the overall goal is to improve the health and quality of life of ageing women by implementing gender-responsive policies, programmes and practices that address the rights, strengths and needs of ageing women throughout the life course. These efforts need to take into account the special situations of older women with disabilities, members of minority groups, those who live in rural areas, and those who have low socioeconomic status.

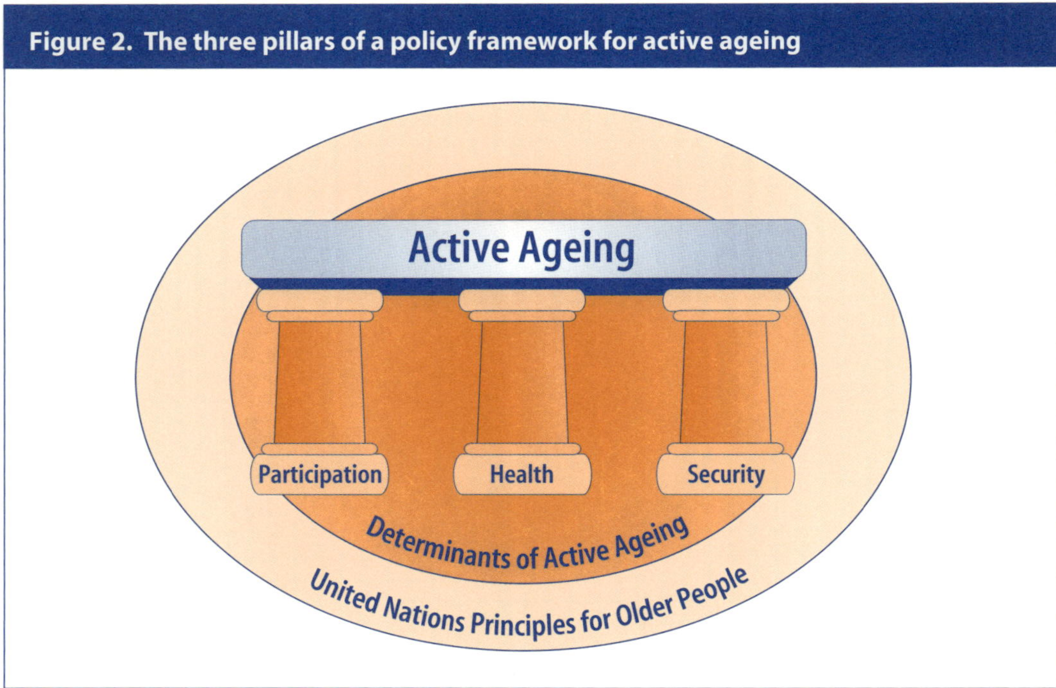

Source: *Active Ageing: A Policy Framework*, WHO, 2002

Fulfilling this goal means that *governments at all levels, international organizations, nongovernmental organizations* and other leaders in *civil society* and the *private sector* need to:

- **mainstream gender and age perspectives** in all policy considerations by taking into account the impact of gender and age-based roles and cultural expectations concerning ageing women's health, participation and security;

- **systematically eliminate inequities based on gender and age** and their interaction with other factors such as race, ethnicity, culture, religion, disability, socioeconomic status and geographic location;

- **acknowledge and address diversity** among older women and men;

- **enable the full and equal participation of older women** and men in the development process and in all economic, social, cultural and spiritual spheres of community life;

- **adopt a life course perspective** that understands ageing and cumulative disadvantage as a process that spans the entire lifespan and provides supportive policies and activities at key transition points in a one's life;

- **encourage intergenerational solidarity** and respect between generations.

Gender analysis has become a common policy tool in many settings. This report proposes that policy-makers apply a dual perspective to their decisions — a perspective that takes both gender and age into account (Figure 3).

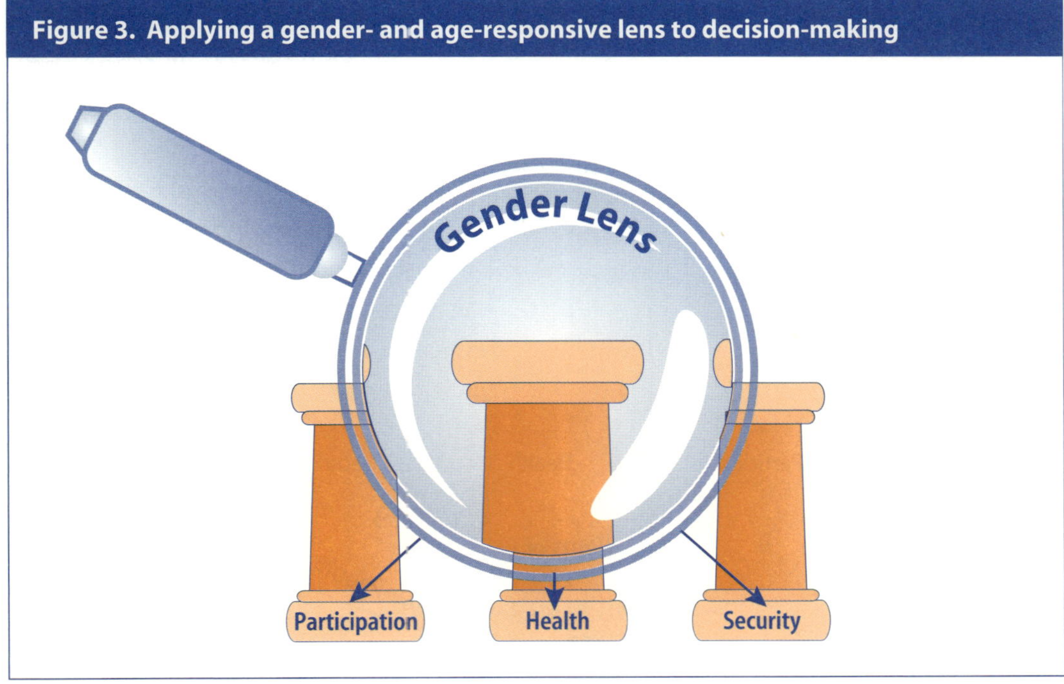

Figure 3. Applying a gender- and age-responsive lens to decision-making

Some questions to ask

Taking gender, age and equity into account

1. Does the policy/programme address gender- and age-specific concerns?

2. Does the policy/programme take gender-, age- and culturally-based traditions and roles into account?

3. Does the available evidence take gender and age differences into account?

4. Does the policy/programme support equity and ensure equal access without discrimination based upon age, gender, class, race, ethnicity, health status, income and place of residence?

Outcomes

5. In what ways does the policy/programme enhance the health/participation/security of older women and older men?

6. How will the policy/programme affect women and men differently throughout the life course, and particularly in older age?

7. Does the policy/programme acknowledge the contribution and strengths of older women and men and the heterogeneity of the older population?

8. Does the policy/programme respect the United Nations Principles for Older People: independence, participation, care, self-fulfillment and dignity?

9. Does the policy/programme support intergenerational solidarity for both women and men and encourage a 'society for all ages'?

10. How have diverse groups of older women and men contributed to the development of the policy or programme?

11. How will the policy/programme be implemented, monitored and evaluated in an age- and gender-responsive way?

An example of how to combine the gender-sensitive/age-friendly lens with the active ageing pillars and determinants is provided in the central pages of this document. It is focused on primary health care services and can be used as a tool to facilitate the identification of issues/concerns; policy/action development; and formulation of research questions.

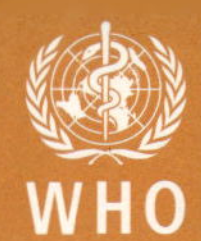

3.   The health status of older women

This chapter provides an overview of the health status of older women. Some diseases and conditions are highlighted in subsequent chapters, and it is therefore important to take all chapters into account when assessing the overall health and well-being of ageing women.

Key points

With a few exceptions, women have longer life expectancies than men in both developed and developing countries. The reasons relate to both female biology such as hormonal protective factors, and fatal risk factors associated with male working conditions, lifestyles and higher risk of injury. Worldwide, women are likely to continue to maintain this advantage over men for the foreseeable future. However, the gender gap in life expectancy is decreasing in some developed countries as a result of role and lifestyle changes such as participation in the paid work force and increased rates of smoking by women.[13,14]

Global inequities in life expectancy among women are immense — for example, a baby girl born in France or Japan can expect to live more than 40 years longer than a baby girl born in a sub-Saharan African country. There are also dramatic differences in women's life expectancy after reaching age 60. For example, a 60-year-old woman in Sierra Leone can expect to live another 14 years while a woman of the same age in Japan can expect to live another 27 years. Mortality patterns also differ within countries; for example, in Australia, Canada and Mexico women in indigenous communities have poorer health and significantly lower life expectancies than non-indigenous women.[15-17] Life expectancy is closely related to income and social status and can vary among neighbourhoods. For example, female life expectancy between women living in London varies from 84.7 years in Kensington/Chelsea to 79 years in Newham. The latter neighbourhood is situated in inner London and is characterized by poor housing conditions, low levels of education and employment, high crime rates and a higher percentage of pensioners living in poverty.[18]

Noncommunicable diseases are the leading cause of death and disability among women in all global regions except Africa.[19] Approximately 80% of chronic disease deaths occur in middle- and low-income countries, where most of the world's ageing women live.

[20]

 For example, studies have shown
that the elevated risk for depression in
women is at least partly accounted for by
negative attitudes towards them, lack of
acknowledgement for their work, fewer opportunities in education and employment,
and greater risk of domestic violence.[21] The
risk of mental illness is also associated with
indicators of poverty, including low levels of
education and, in some studies, with poor
housing and low-income.[22]

[21] Women and men
are equally likely to develop Alzheimer's
disease and other dementias in old age;
however, the prevalence is higher among
women because they live longer.[23] The
emotional, social and financial costs of
Alzheimer disease to families and societies are already massive and will continue to
increase.[23,24] Worldwide, older people have
a higher risk of completed suicide than any
other age group. The male:female ratio for
completed suicides among people over age
75 is 3:1 to 4:1.[25]

[26,27] Depression may also be secondary to a medical disorder or to use of medi-
cation use. Women are approximately twice
as likely as men to experience a depressive
episode within their lifetimes.[23] It is estimated that by the year 2020, depression
will be the second most important cause of
disability burden in the world.[28]

 The
impact of communicable diseases such as
malaria, tuberculosis and leprosy grows
increasingly severe with time and ageing.
For example, an individual who experienced pulmonary tuberculosis early in life
may – even if successfully treated – sustain
residual ventilatory incapacity which can
be aggravated by the ageing process in later
years. In all countries, older people are at
high risk for contracting influenza and its
complications, including death.

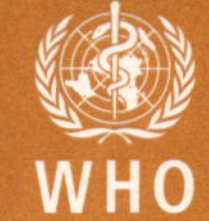

Ageing women remain at risk for HIV/AIDS and other sexually transmitted infections (STIs). Like ageing men, women can remain sexually active until the end of life, but they may have fewer opportunities because most outlive their partners. Many STIs are physically transmitted more efficiently at all ages from males to females than from females to males. The risk is increased by customs such as older men engaging in extramarital relationships, widow cleansing, polygamy and wife inheritance, as well as by older women's roles as caregivers. Once infected, women face a disproportionate burden of sequelae from STIs, including AIDS resulting from HIV infection and cervical cancer as a result of the transmission of the human papilloma virus (HPV).

The HIV/AIDS epidemic has had devastating economic, social, health and psychological impacts on older women especially in sub-Saharan Africa. Older women care for those who are ill with HIV/AIDS and then for their orphaned children, and are themselves at risk of infection. Studies show that older caregivers are under severe financial, physical and emotional stress — including arising from financial hardships leading to inability to pay for food, clothing, essential drugs and basic health care; a lack of information about self-protection while providing care to their infected children and grandchildren; stigmatization of people with the disease; negative attitudes of health workers towards them as older persons, as well as towards people living with HIV/AIDS; and physical and emotional stress resulting from increasing levels of violence and abuse.[29,30]

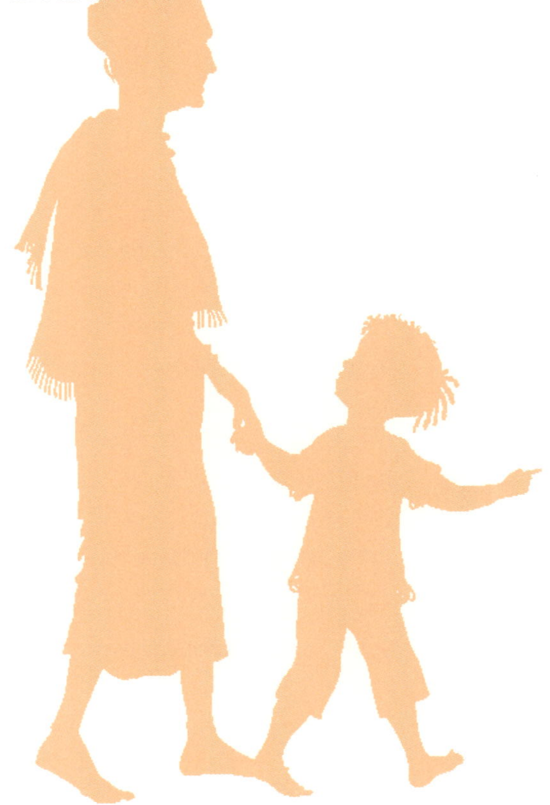

Heart disease and stroke are significant causes of death and disability in women in both developed and developing countries[19] and especially among women who are poor.[31] Hormone replacement therapy, which was widely used in high-income countries has been shown not to prevent heart disease after menopause as was originally thought, but rather is associated with an increased risk of stroke and heart disease among some ageing women.[32,33] Women with heart disease tend to present with different symptoms than men and are less likely to seek or to be provided with medical help and to be properly diagnosed until late in the disease process. While improvements have been made, women are less likely to have access to appropriate investigations and treatment, and are more likely to be underrepresented in research on heart disease.[34]

The lifetime risk for breast cancer among women in most developed countries is about one in ten. This risk increases with age – especially after age 50 – and only declines after the age of 80. Lower fertility rates, increasing age of pregnancy and a decrease in the number of years of breastfeeding all contribute to a predicted rise in breast cancer in developing countries.

Cervical cancer, which kills an estimated 239,000 women every year is – after cancers of the stomach and breast – the third most common cancer in women in developing countries. Providing girls with a new vaccine to prevent infection from the human papilloma virus (HPV), which causes cervical cancer, offers the possibility of eliminating the incidence of cervical cancer in the future. Meanwhile, it is critical to provide existing cohorts of ageing women with pap smear screening or other low-cost prevention and screening technologies.[35] Use of these techniques can dramatically reduce mortality due to cervical cancer.

Osteoarthritis and osteoporosis are associated with chronic pain, limited quality of life and disability. Between the ages of 60 and 90 years, the incidence of osteoarthritis rises 20-fold in women as compared to 10-fold in men.[36] Osteoporosis is three times more common in women than in men, partly because women have a lower peak bone mass and partly because of the hormonal changes that occur at menopause and the effect of pregnancy which can alter calcium composition in a woman's body in the absence of appropriate diet and/or administration of calcium supplements. While these diseases and consequent fractures, spontaneous or caused by falls, place an enormous burden on the health care system and society, often they do not get the attention they deserve because they are incorrectly seen as an inevitable part of ageing or less serious than such conditions as heart disease or cancer.

NOTE: Lung cancer, diabetes and osteoporosis are discussed in subsequent chapters.

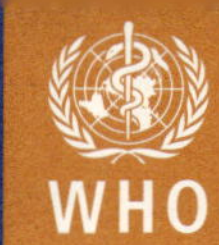

Implications for policy, practice and research

Life expectancy. While life expectancy is a crude measure of health, it does provide the ultimate yardstick. Efforts to overcome dramatic inequities in life expectancies among older women between countries, and among various socioeconomic population sub-groups within a given country or region, must become an international priority.

Preventing noncommunicable diseases. While the progression from mortality caused by infectious diseases to that caused by chronic diseases is a positive sign of improvements in public health, the increase in chronic diseases due to population ageing has substantial implications for human suffering and health care costs. The ultimate goal is to prevent and manage chronic diseases, thus postponing disability and death and enabling ageing women and men to maintain their positive contributions to society. If this achievement is to be shared equally by women and men, policies and programmes must take both gender and age into account.

Addressing inequities in diseases that affect older women. Tackling inequities in ***coronary heart disease*** requires the education and training of health professionals about sex and gender differences in the clinical manifestations and progress of the disease, the full inclusion of older women in cardiac studies, earlier and more aggressive control of risk factors, and appropriate access to diagnosis and treatment.[34]

In light of the high burden of ***breast cancer***, and predictions that the incidence will increase worldwide, there remains an urgent need for a better understanding of its root causes, increased availability of effective and affordable screening tools for use with older women, the expansion of effective treatment regimes, and support for breast cancer survivors.

Use of the new vaccine to prevent HPV infection must be made widely available immediately in low-income countries where ***cervical cancer*** is a major cause of death. For older women, the use of pap smears and other cost-effective prevention and treatment technologies must be made universally available.

Health care priorities need to redress the imbalance in attention given to musculoskeletal disorders and joint diseases such as ***osteoporosis and arthritis***.

Another inequity that needs to be addressed involves ***blindness***. Local initiatives and the political will to eliminate gender inequities in eye care services are critical steps in achieving the goals of Vision 2020, a global initiative to combat avoidable blindness.

A gender-sensitive approach to improving mental health. Understanding that mental health and mental illness are the results of complex interactions among biological, psychological, and sociocultural factors is important for those considering ageing women. Such understanding places mental health and illness within the social context of women's life experiences and implies that equality and social justice are important goals for improving mental well-being among women of all ages. Developing gender-sensitive national policies, with budgets dedicated to mental health and mental illness, needs to become a priority in all countries. Evidence suggests that practices and programmes encouraging socialization and physical activity can help ease depression, [37,38] and that most mental health problems in later life can be dealt with in age-friendly primary health care services, and through community services and interventions that support families and caregivers. [39,40]

Communicable diseases. Older women will be major beneficiaries of efforts to control and eliminate infectious diseases in settings where communicable diseases are common. WHO urges all Member States to implement a national influenza vaccination policy and to implement strategies to increase vaccination coverage of all people at high risk, with the goal of attaining coverage of the older population of at least 50% by 2006 and 75% by 2010. [41]

HIV/AIDS and other STIs. It is essential to dispel the myth that older women are not sexually active. Sexual health care, education and knowledge about STIs and HIV/ AIDS are important not only for women of reproductive age but also for girls and women in all stages of life. This concept needs to be considered when allocating resources and planning future research and programming. Programmes and prevention messages must be sex- and age-specific and should target not only individual behaviours but also the social and cultural context in which these behaviours occur.

The participation and representation of older people – and older women in particular – in HIV/AIDS programme planning at local, district and national levels will improve the response to HIV/AIDS. This response will require support to older people and their organizations. Health care staff should be appropriately trained to support older people who are infected and appropriate drugs should be made available as recommended by the WHO universal access approach.

Dissemination of research and information. There are few controlled studies on depression in older women. [28] Similarly, gender-specific research into the causes and management of dementia becomes increasingly critical as life expectancies increase. Because of the stigma attached to suicide in many cultures, it is likely that the number of suicides among older men and women are undercounted. Many questions about suicide in later life remain unanswered.

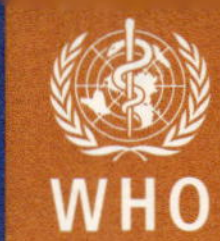

Table 1. Life expectancy at birth and at age 60, women, selected countries, 2006									
	At birth	At age 60		At birth	At age 60		At birth	At age 60
AFRO			**EURO**			**SEARO**		
Mozambique	46	16	Bulgaria	76	20	India	63	18
Senegal	57	17	Russian Federation	72	19	Indonesia	69	18
Sierra Leone	40	14				Sri Lanka	77	21
			Switzerland	83	26			
AMRO			**EMRO**			**WPRO**		
Brazil	74	22				China	74	20
			Bahrain	75	20			
Canada	83	25				Japan	86	27
			Egypt	70	18			
Haiti	56	17				Papua New Guinea	61	14
			Pakistan	63	17			

Source: World Health Report, 2006.

Further studies are needed on the sex and gender-linked factors that contribute to lung cancer, breast cancer, heart disease and obesity.

Currently, older people are largely invisible in international data on HIV/AIDS infection rates because data collection does not routinely include the over-50 age group.

There is a critical need for improved surveillance and for the collection of sex- and age-specific data after age 50. Also needed are controlled trials on the epidemiology, pathogenesis, and therapeutic and clinical outcomes of older HIV-infected patients.

4. Health and social services

In order to be comprehensive, health systems should provide a continuum of gender-responsive care from promotion and prevention to acute and palliative care, as well as access to essential medications.

Key points

 For example, in many countries, older women are less likely than men to receive cataract surgery and *eye care* due to the cost of examinations, eyeglasses, drops and surgery, as well as gender- and age-discrimination, and a lack of support for and information about treatment.[20] Men may gain quicker access to *selective operations*[42,43] and a life-saving procedure following a heart attack.[44,45, 46] These inequities may be a result of direct or indirect gender- and age-based discrimination, older women's lower financial status and limited access to health security schemes, and a focus on reproductive health that excludes older women.

From a global perspective, the use of medications can be a double-edged sword. In most countries, older women who have low incomes and no access to benefits covering the costs of medications either go without or spend a large part of their meager incomes on drugs. In contrast, medications are sometimes overprescribed to older women who have insurance or the means to pay for medications. Older women may be more likely than men to experience adverse drug reactions because of smaller body size, altered body metabolism and diminished ability to compensate for drug-induced changes in normal homeostasis.[47]

The barriers to primary health care faced by older people are often worse for older women. These barriers include lack of transportation, low literacy levels and a lack of money to pay for services and medications. Invariably, gender and age interact with socioeconomic status, race and ethnicity. For example, older women who are homeless or do not speak the dominant language may have even less access to health care and be more likely to encounter discrimination in treatment.

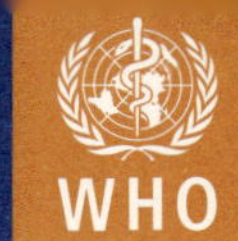

Personal expenses related to health care gradually take up a greater share of a woman's resources as she grows older, even in highly industrialized countries. For example, studies in the United States of America (USA) show that health security is out of reach for many women over the age of 50, and that out-of-pocket expenses for medications and long-term care are major factors contributing to higher poverty rates among older women.[48] Because women most often work at home or in the informal sector or part-time, they have limited or no access to health insurance schemes that are tied to employment.

Because women live longer than men and are more likely to be alone in old age, policy-makers and practitioners must pay special attention to the gender implications of long-term care policies and programmes, whether they be in the community or in residential facilities. Most long-term care for older people who cannot live independently is provided by informal support systems such as family members and neighbours. But as the number of very old women continues to increase and the pool of available caregivers continues to decrease, families and policy makers will increasingly need to look for other options. Part of the answer may lie in increased home and community support services, but it is likely that the number of very old women who spend their last years in institutional settings will also increase.

Palliative end-of-life care in the home or in small hospices will become increasingly important to health systems as the number of very old women and men continues to increase. Services include pain relief, and medical, spiritual and psychological support to the dying person and her family, as well as respite care for burdened caregivers.

Home caregivers (who are mostly middle-aged and older women) of people who are ill must be supported and nurtured to enable them to maximize the care they deliver, to manage the considerable stress that can accompany caregiving, and to be able to sustain a caregiving role over a long period of time — often many years. Poor families are in particularly precarious positions and – as more and more women work outside the home – a better balance in the sharing of caregiving between women and men becomes increasingly important.[49]

In both developed and developing countries, a range of health care reforms has had a negative effect on women, particularly in middle- and older age.[50] User fees and private provider schemes limit access to services for older women.[51,52] The closing of acute-care beds, and early release from hospital without a corresponding increase in support in the community, leaves ageing women with an increased and unrecognized burden of caring for partners and other family members who are ill or frail.

Implications for policy, practice and research

Health professionals. Professionals need to understand and recognize sex and age differences — especially when prescribing medications, treating mental health problems such as depression, and dealing with health problems related to domestic abuse. A gender perspective means going beyond physical symptoms to explore the socio-cultural as well as the biological factors underlying these problems.

Medications. The goal is to ensure equity in the provision of essential, and high-quality drugs among all age groups and between women and men. At the same time, physicians and pharmacists need to take into account the risks of overprescribing medications based upon gender stereotyping, and of the adverse effects of multiple drug use among older women.

Supporting informal care. The needs of caregivers are confounded by culture, income, living arrangements and the extent of support from others. Caregivers of people who are ill or frail need information about specific conditions, treatment, medications, warning symptoms and necessary lifestyle modifications. They need training in home health skills and how to work in partnership with health care providers. Equally important are skills to help them identify available resources, navigate the system and become effective advocates for recipients

of care. Caregivers also need a forum to express their experiences and recommendations for system change and for sensitizing service providers. Most importantly, caregivers need "respite"— time off from their caregiving role.

Some of the options for financially supporting caregivers include leave from work (paid and unpaid), tax policies and payments for caregiving services. In developing countries it is especially important to foster intergenerational relationships and co-residency by providing subsidies for those who care for older relatives, housing designs that enable multigenerational living, and community centres that can be used by older people as meeting places and clubs.[53]

Health care reform. Cost-cutting measures must not expect to transfer formal care to the unremunerated care provided by ageing women without providing compensation for lost wages and community support services. Priority setting in health care services should be based on evidence that is free from systematic gender- and age- biases.

Health security. The goal is to provide equal access to essential health services and medications, regardless of ability to pay. Because older women have fewer financial resources to pay for services and private insurance premiums, taxes and social insurance schemes that are not based on time spent in formal employment provide the most equitable basis for health financing. Health insurance schemes should ensure that vulnerable and marginalized groups, including older women are adequately covered.

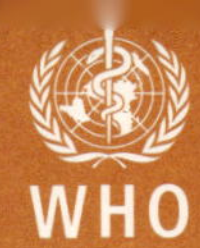

Mental health services. Policies and practices that benefit older women and men should:

- support and improve the care provided by their families (e.g. respite care, training);

- incorporate mental health assessment and management of depression as well as other mental health problems into primary health care;

- pay special attention to women who have experienced elder abuse or other forms of violence ;

- help to remove the stigma associated with mental illness; and

- include legislation to protect the human rights of institutionalized people with severe mental disorders.

Cataract surgical coverage

Cataract is the leading cause of visual impairment in all regions of the world, except in the most developed countries.[54] In many countries, older women with cataracts are much less likely to have surgery than men — a classic example of how gender bias impacts on access to health services.[20]

Research and information dissemination. Priority areas for developing and sharing knowledge include:

- ways to increase access to primary health care and participation in health promotion and disease prevention activities particularly among older women in minority groups, who have low socio-economic status and who live in rural and isolated areas;

- cost-effective ways to help older women remain in their homes in the community;

- gender perspectives, expectations and experiences of long-term care options;

- effective policy options and legal guidelines for providing dignified long-term and end-of-life care to older women and men;

- more detailed evidence on the differential use of medications by older women and men and whether gender is systematically associated with inappropriate use;

- best practices related to receiving and giving care (i.e. filial, state and personal responsibilities); and

- the impact of health care reform on gender equity.

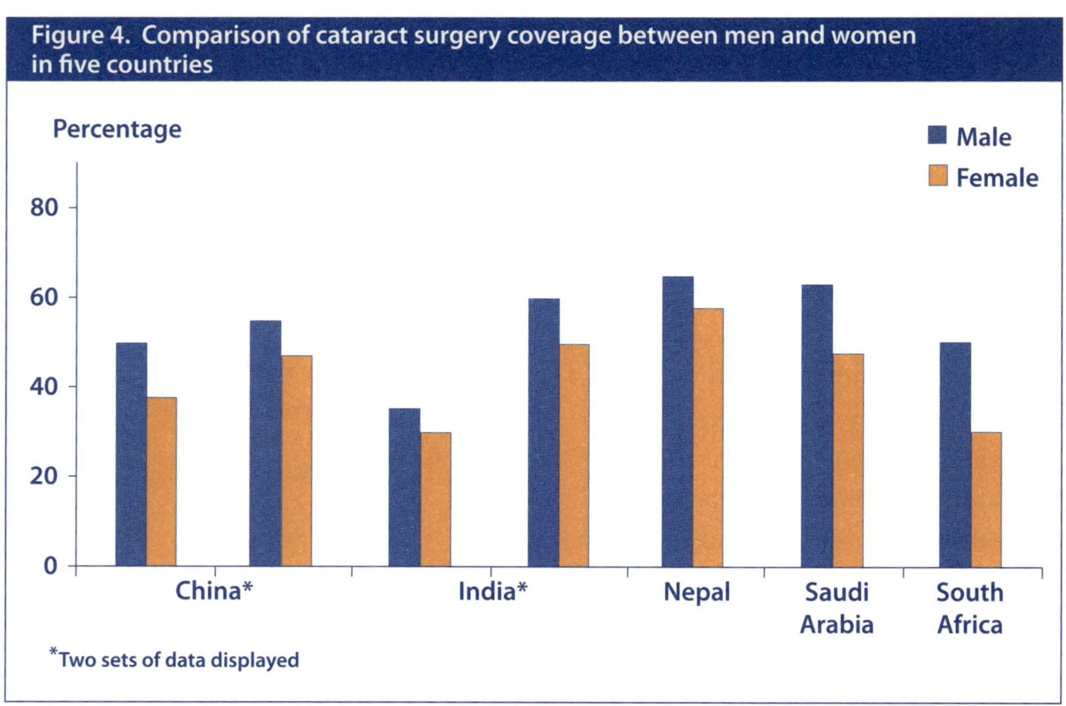

Figure 4. Comparison of cataract surgery coverage between men and women in five countries

Source: Lewallen S. and Courtright P. British Columbia Centre for Epidemiologic and International Ophthalmology. *Gender and use of cataract surgical services in developing countries.* Vancouver: University of British Columbia, 2000 (unpublished paper).

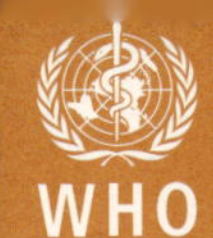

5. Personal determinants

Biology and genetics

Although biology and genetics are key determinants of women's health, the evidence suggests that most of the time other factors related to gender-influenced roles and status are more important in determining the health and well-being of women at midlife and older ages. However, as is the case with all the determinants of active ageing, sex and gender are likely to interact in synergistic ways.

Key points

It has been estimated that only 20-25% of variability in the age at death is explained by genetic factors.[55] The influence of genetic factors on the development of chronic conditions varies significantly. For example, some women have a genetic predisposition to breast and ovarian cancer; even when this risk is known, however, it is not a foregone conclusion that they will develop the disease in their lifetime.

While women are more likely to survive into older age, they have more disability than men in every age group after age 60, as well as more co-morbidities.[56-58] Biological factors may be a critical reason for this. For example, lower levels of muscle strength and bone density in women increase the likelihood of disabling conditions such as frailty and osteoporosis, and difficulty with tasks requiring optimal threshold levels of strength. However, the incidence and prevalence of disability is also influenced by socioeconomic conditions, and gender-based discrimination. For example, women may have had inadequate access to nutritious food in early life. As another example, in some cultures restrictions on movement outside the home are placed upon widows.

Normal ageing includes some natural declines and physiological changes that lead to a loss of functional capacity and reserve. These include reductions in hearing and vision capacities, a decrease in taste, smell and thirst sensations, and declines in basal metabolic rate and immunological response. There is also a significant reduction in bone density and muscle mass, both of which are more pronounced in women than in men.[59,60] However, individuals may experience these declines at very different rates. Physiological declines associated with ageing will likely be exaggerated for a woman who has lived a life of poverty with poor nutrition and has had little, if any, access to education and health care.

For ageing women, menopause is a significant transition from both a biological and social perspective. Hormonal changes occurring during the menopausal period are related – either directly or indirectly – to adverse effects on quality of life, body composition and cardiovascular risk. Women's advantage over men in terms of cardiovascular disease gradually disappears with the significant declines in estrogen levels after menopause. The loss of bone density at menopause is a significant reason why women have much higher rates of osteoporosis than men.[61]

Menopause is directly associated with physical symptoms including increases in vasomotor symptoms, vaginal dryness, pain during sexual intercourse, and central abdominal fat, as well as decreases in breast tenderness, bone mineral density and sexual functioning. Mood, self-rated condition of health, and life satisfaction are not directly related to the menopause transition. There is no evidence that memory loss or dementia is linked to menopause.[62]

Hormone replacement therapy (HRT) has not been found to be effective in preventing heart disease but rather is associated with an increased risk of heart disease, stroke, and breast cancer. Generally, the use of HRT is now only recommended in low doses for short periods of time to deal with severe symptoms such as vaginal atrophy and hot flashes that prevent sleeping. This therapy may be especially important for women who undergo an early and dramatic menopause due to surgical interventions.[63]

Women's experience of living through the menopausal period is dramatically affected by sociocultural factors. The most relevant factors influencing a woman's quality of life during the menopause transition appear to be her previous emotional and physical health, her social situation, her experience of stressful life events, and the beliefs about menopause and female ageing in her culture.[64] For all women, leaving the reproductive years marks both an important change and a window for growth. Regardless of differences in how it is experienced, the menopausal transition can provide an important focus, a time that can be used to reassess one's health, lifestyle and goals.

There are indications of intergenerational factors in obesity, such as parental obesity, maternal gestational diabetes, and maternal birth weight. Interactions between early and later factors throughout the life course can be particularly harmful in later years. For example, low birth weight followed by adult obesity has been shown to result in a significantly higher risk for cardiovascular disease.[65]

Reduced muscle mass (sarcopenia) in older age can have significant consequences for day-to-day living. For example, the Framingham study showed that 40% of women aged 55 to 64 and 65% of women aged 75 to 84 were unable to lift 4.5 kilograms.[66]

Biological factors that relate to reproduction have traditionally been the major focus of policies and programmes related to women's health. Research and health care practices that focus almost exclusively on women's reproductive biology fail to address chronic diseases and the broad social determinants of active ageing that lead to health or illness as women grow older.

Implications for policy, practice and research: biology and genetics

Health Services. While high-quality, accessible reproductive health services remain critical to women's well-being, health services need to expand beyond a focus on reproductive biology and adjust to today's realities of an ageing population. This must include age- and gender-sensitive services geared to the prevention and management of chronic diseases such as heart disease, diabetes, arthritis, and Alzheimer disease.

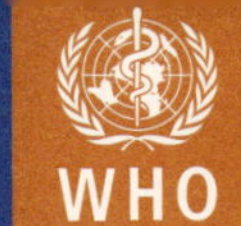

Disability. A focus on healthy, active ageing and improved health services can lead to the compression of morbidity and disabilities until very late in life. At the same time, the dramatic increase in the number of older women in both developed and developing countries will inevitably lead to an overall increase in the number of older women with disabilities. To improve older women's quality of life and to keep health care costs down, more attention needs to be paid to preventing and managing disabilities.

Preventing problems associated with biological ageing. Regular physical activity, healthy eating and not smoking can prevent and alleviate problems associated with age-related loss of muscle strength and bone density and of increases in fat mass. Governments and civil society need to overcome ageist attitudes that suggest these healthy lifestyle behaviours are not important or appropriate for older women.

Dispelling misconceptions about menopause. Policies and programmes need to dispel misconceptions about the menopausal period and encourage ageing women to adopt healthy lifestyle behaviours (such as healthy eating and regular physical activity) that will help them cope with the physical symptoms of menopause.

Research and information dissemination. The burden of disability in older women has wide-ranging and profound effects on older women themselves, their families, and the health care system. Gender-sensitive trials aimed at prevention of disability in older age should be considered a priority in the allocation of resources for health and social care research. This work needs to take a life course perspective that underscores the gender-related factors in the physical, social and economic environments that are associated with women's disabilities in later life.

More cross-cultural knowledge about menopause is needed. Other knowledge needs relate to the perimenopausal period — especially among women who experience severe symptoms during this time or as a result of either an early but natural or surgery-induced menopause. Other priorities include gathering evidence about alternative therapies and lifestyle changes to deal with the concerns of menopause, and the relationship between hormonal changes after menopause and chronic diseases such as heart disease.

Psychological and spiritual factors

Psychological capacities that are acquired across the life course greatly influence the way in which people age. Self-efficacy (the belief people have in their capacity to exert control over their lives), optimism, and a sense of coherence are linked to mental and social well-being as one ages. Coping styles determine how well people adapt to the transitions (such as retirement) and negative life events associated with ageing (such as bereavement and the onset of illness).[67] There is some evidence in developing countries that ageing women are more resilient than men when it comes to later life transitions and coping with crises.[68]

Active ageing also depends on a person's ability to maintain meaning in life despite personal losses, physical decline and ageism. While worldwide studies on gender differences are lacking, North American studies show that current cohorts of older women, and particularly those in minority races and ethnic groups rely heavily on prayer and faith as a way to cope with losses associated with ageing.[69] For many older people, spirituality and/or religion provides much of this meaning.

Besides offering hope in the face of death, faith can provide consolation and strength during difficult times, and a guide for daily living. Being a valued member of a congregation of believers also is a source of social support and of self-esteem.[70] Pastoral care and counselling may be particularly important to older women at the end of life who are alone and unable to leave their homes due to severe disabilities.

In addition to supporting an older woman in her search for spiritual answers, faith institutions and religious groups can be an important source of social support, validation, hope and reassurance that her life and death have meaning. However, negative practices such as harmful mourning rites for widows that are associated with religious rituals in some cultures are damaging to older women's health.

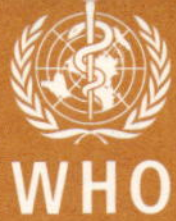

6. Behavioural determinants

Much of the physical decline that occurs with ageing is related to health behaviours including poor nutrition, physical inactivity, smoking, and a failure to use preventive services.

Key points

Young girls are now smoking at least as much – if not more – than young boys.[71] Moreover, while tobacco use has declined in some high-income countries, it is increasing in some low- and middle-income countries — especially among young people and women. This trend is predicted to increase, at least partly because of changing norms towards women's roles combined with pervasive, gender-specific advertising by the tobacco industry.[72] The tobacco industry targets girls and young women using false images of vitality, slimness, sophistication, sexual allure, and autonomy.[71]

While tobacco causes similar health problems for men and women, it poses some additional threats in ageing women. These threats include an increased risk of cardiovascular disease and bone fractures due to reduced bone mass.[71] There is conclusive evidence that the effects of smoking on women include pre-cancerous changes of the cervix, and cervical cancer, which is the leading cause of cancer in women worldwide. Some studies have shown that women who smoke are more likely to experience certain menopausal symptoms such as hot flashes, night sweats and insomnia as well as early menopause.[73]

Increases in smoking among women, and gender-related roles in the household have led to a fourfold increase in the incidence of lung cancer among women over the last 30 years. The increase in lung cancer in the USA and several other countries has led to it overtaking breast cancer as the leading cause of cancer death in women. Most of this is due to increased smoking by women. However, women's risk for lung cancer is also elevated by gender-related roles and positions in the household. Many women who do not smoke but live with husbands who do are exposed to second-hand tobacco smoke. In their role of preparing food, many women in poor countries are exposed to fumes and smoke from solid cooking fuels, which also exacerbate their vulnerability to lung cancer.[74-77]

Generally, as people age, their activity levels tend to decrease; older women are less active than older men, at least in terms of deliberate exercise (they may be more active than men in everyday chores).[78,79] Barriers to activity for ageing women include cost and access, lack of time due to work and family responsibilities, disparities in income and education, cultural restrictions, a lack of social support (including inadequate counselling by physicians) and low self-efficacy (for example, feeling less physically competent).[80]

Compelling evidence links physical activity with healthy ageing, such as improvements in physical and mental health, as well as disease prevention and control, enhanced emotional and social well-being, improved mobility and balance, and increased autonomy and independence. Older women who are active are at lower risk of osteoporosis, cardiovascular disease, obesity, back pain, and falls.[78] Physical activity may also be an antidote to the unpleasant side effects of menopause experienced by some women and can help prevent or reduce the weight gain and the increases in abdominal fat that often accompany middle-age.[81]

Healthy eating enhances resistance to diseases such as cancer, promotes optimal brain functioning, and helps prevent osteoporosis and other chronic health problems. There is some evidence that the incidence rate of atherosclerotic disease is significantly less in women who eat 5-10 servings of fruit and vegetables per day compared with those who eat 2-5 servings.[82] Because of increased risk for low bone density after menopause, older women need increased calcium intake and regular weight-bearing activity.[83] Vitamin D is also essential for both bone and muscle strength. Serious deficiency of vitamin D is common among those who are housebound or in nursing homes and long stay wards, and has been identified as an important public health problem.[84]

Once considered as solely as a problem for developed countries, rates of obesity are climbing quickly in developing countries as the availability of foods that are affordable and high in fat and sugar increases worldwide and people adopt more sedentary lifestyles. The number of older people who are overweight (those whose body mass index is 25 or above) and obese (body mass index above 30) has increased dramatically in recent years. For example, among adults aged 60-69 in selected cities in Latin America and the Caribbean, 61% are overweight and among these about half are obese.[85] This trend is projected to continue unless dramatic steps are taken. The largest increase is projected to be among women from upper middle-income countries.[86]

Among ageing women, obesity increases susceptibility to a number of diseases and chronic conditions such as endometrial cancer and gallbladder disease, and may encumber mobility by exacerbating conditions such as osteoarthritis, which is more common in women than in men. Obesity puts women at greater risk of developing diabetes than men. Often, low socioeconomic status is linked to a higher risk of obesity and to developing diabetes.

Type 2 diabetes, which is closely associated with obesity, can be prevented by weight control and physical activity. Studies in China, Finland, and the USA have shown that even a moderate reduction in weight and only half an hour of walking each day reduced the incidence of diabetes by more than one half.[87]

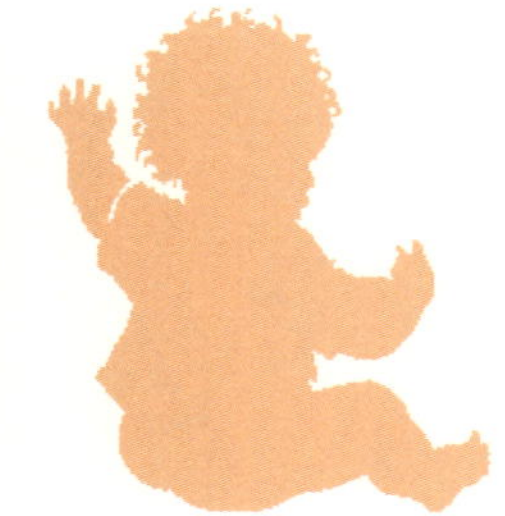

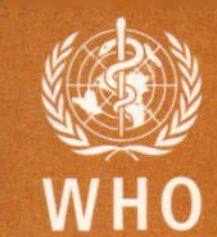

Obesity and a lack of exercise are major contributors to urinary incontinence, which is two to three times higher among older women than among older men. In old age, incontinence is a predictor of the loss of independence and a key factor in institutionalization. Other causes of incontinence, especially in developing countries include frequent childbirth, poor repair of birth injuries, and untreated urinary tract infections. In these situations, improved reproductive health in younger women is the best way to prevent incontinence problems in old age.

Available evidence clearly indicates that healthy lifestyle practices such as nutritious eating, regular physical activity, not smoking and moderate or no alcohol use as proactive, non-prescription approaches are effective in dealing with the symptoms of menopause. Many women also use a variety of supplements and alternative medicines made from plants, although the efficacy and safety of these are still inconclusive.

Diabetes

Approximately 176 million people have diabetes mellitus worldwide and this number may well double by the year 2025.[87] Differences in prevalence vary between women and men, and between countries and regions. For example, in Latin America and the Caribbean, the female prevalence of diabetes and obesity is approximately 15 to 20% higher than that for males.[85] Overall in Canada, men have higher rates of diabetes than women, although the sub-population with the highest rates is Aboriginal women.[88] Women who developed impaired glucose tolerance during pregnancy (gestational diabetes) are at greater risk of developing diabetes later in life if they become overweight. Diabetes greatly accelerates atherosclerosis, more in women than in men.[89] In the early stages of Type 2 diabetes, the disease is mostly asymptomatic which is one reason why so many cases remain undiagnosed. In later stages, it can lead to diabetic ulcers and gangrene requiring amputation and kidney failure.

Implications for policy, practice and research

Increased attention to health promotion.
Women are never too old to benefit from health promotion and self-care initiatives that encourage them to remain socially active, engage in regular physical activity, maintain a healthy weight, and refrain from behaviours that could have a detrimental effect on their health, such as smoking, excessive drinking and overeating. Those approaches that promote self-empowerment and peer-leadership are most likely to be effective.

While health promotion and prevention efforts should start early in life, programmes should also be available to older women and men. Physicians, nurses and other health- and social-service workers need to learn how to advise older people to quit smoking, drink alcohol in moderation or not at all, eat in a healthy way and stay physically active. Social marketing campaigns can help dispel erroneous beliefs about eating, smoking, and exercising in older age.

Guidelines and education. Culturally appropriate, and gender-responsive guidelines for healthy eating and physical activity, and which are specific to older people should be developed and taught in the community. These guidelines should include gender-specific needs such as increased calcium and vitamin D for women during and after menopause.

Making the healthy choices the easy choices.
Policies related to income, dental care, education, housing and other social factors affect personal health behaviours. Age- and gender-specific interventions that address underlying cultural values, practices and opportunities in the physical environment are needed to make the healthy choices the easy choices. For example, older women who are confined by cultural traditions, or who are housebound looking after an ailing spouse, have few or no opportunities to engage in physical activity. Older women who do not readily have accessible transportation may be unable to purchase fruits and vegetables and calcium-rich foods unless a market or shop is nearby.

Heading off the tobacco-related disease epidemic among ageing women. In most countries, some form of government action (including taxes and legislation) has been enacted to control tobacco consumption and mitigate exposure to second-hand smoke. Countries that have adopted comprehensive tobacco control strategies and policies that address prevention, protection, and cessation have seen considerable success.[90] These efforts must address gender- and age-specific risks.

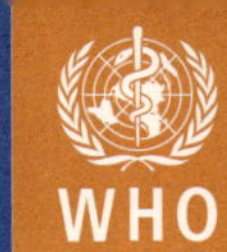

Research and information dissemination.
Policy and programme research is needed
to determine how best to stop the spread of
cigarette smoking to women in countries
where their smoking rates are still fairly
low. Another important question is how
best to remove barriers, and to enable older
women in all countries and varied cultures
to become and stay more physically active.
Other priority areas for developing and
sharing knowledge include how to overcome cultural barriers to healthy living
faced by older women, and the role of exercise, smoking cessation and healthy eating
(including alternative and complementary
supplements) in ameliorating hot flashes
and other conditions associated with the
menopausal period. There is significant

controversy over optimal weights for older
women and whether body mass index
(BMI) measurements are appropriate for
older adults given that weight is distributed
differently (i.e. less muscle, more fat) as we
age. This area requires further sex- and age-
specific exploration.

As this graph shows, the incidence of lung
cancer mortality has increased in women
over the past thirty years in most developed
countries. At the same time, the death rate
for men has declined in countries such as
Australia and the United Kingdom where
men took up smoking earlier than women
and have quit smoking in greater numbers
over the last 20 years.

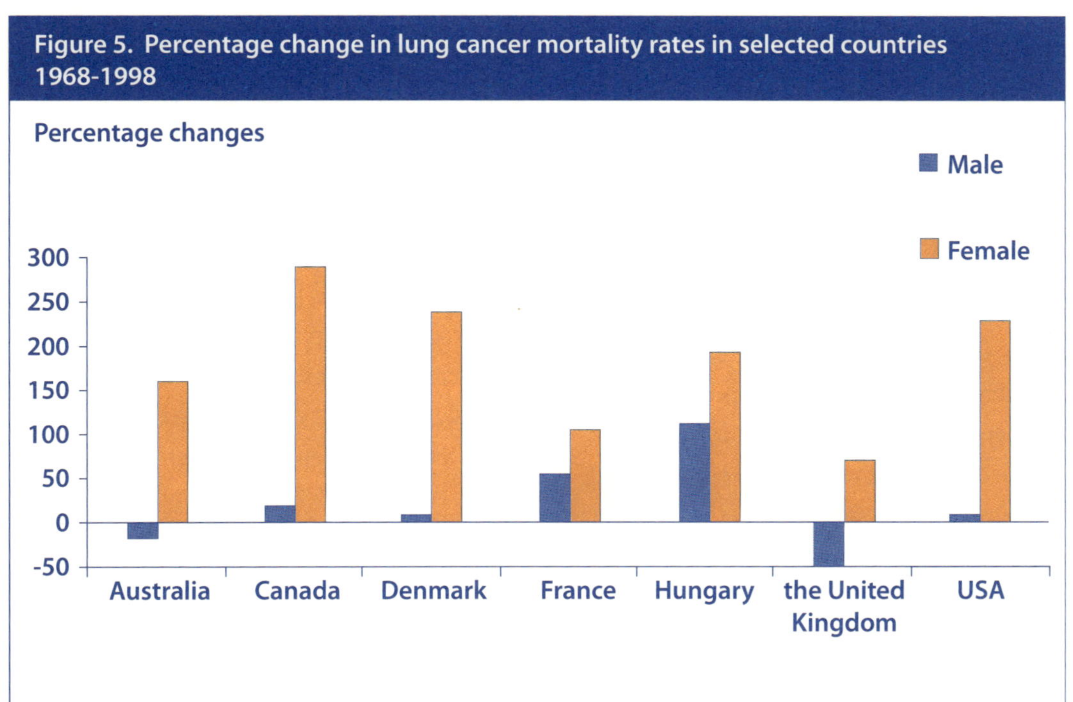

Figure 5. Percentage change in lung cancer mortality rates in selected countries 1968-1998

Source: Parkin D. M. et al. Globoscan (2000). *Cancer incidence, mortality and prevalence worldwide. Version 1.01. 2001.*

7. Economic determinants

Key points

Ageing women make an important contribution to the socioeconomic well-being of their families, communities and nations. Much of this is unpaid and unrecognized work in caregiving, child-rearing, domestic and volunteer occupations. A Swiss study calculated the economic value of family care work to be between 10 and 12 billion Swiss francs, exceeding the cumulative spending on both home-care services and residential care homes.[91] In Africa and other areas hard hit by the HIV/AIDS pandemic and the migration of men and young women in a search of jobs, older women are increasingly serving as the financial and emotional heads of households.[92]

The greatest threat to ageing women's health is poverty. Poverty compromises older women's access to food, shelter, health care, social inclusion and dignity. Women of all ages make up 70% of the world's 1.3 billion very poor — those who live on the equivalent of less than US$1 per day[93] and poverty is often worsened in old age. The vast majority live in the developing world where rapid ageing has not been accompanied by the increase in wealth experienced by industrialized countries. In all countries, some groups of women are especially vulnerable to poverty: older women who are widowed or divorced, women with disabilities, those who are looking after AIDS orphans, grandchildren and other family members, refugees and immigrants, and women in visible minority and indigenous groups.

Even in high-income countries, relative poverty and income inequities have a detrimental effect on well-being, functioning and personal health behaviours.[12] In some developed countries, recent increases in the gap between rich and poor have hit older women hard. In the United Kingdom for example, the *2003 Labour Force Survey* showed that one in four single women pensioners lived in poverty and twice as many women as men relied on means-tested benefits in retirement.[94]

Discrimination in wages, employment, and pension policies hurts older women. Those women, who make up a large pool of workers in the informal economy (e.g. agriculture and petty trading), work until very old age in precarious jobs that have no social security schemes or health care benefits. Older women are increasingly employed in the formal workforce, mostly in low paying and part-time jobs. All over the world, women have lower labour force participation rates, higher unemployment and significant pay differences. Women earn less than men, even when they have comparable education and training.[93] Most significantly, women's earning power is interrupted by pregnancy, childrearing and (in mid- and later life) caregiving responsibilities. This means that even the small proportion of older women who are eligible for pensions because they were employed in the formal sector, receive lower benefits than men.

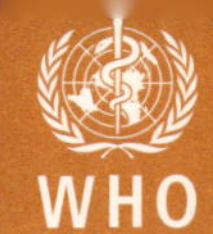

Undernutrition and older women

Undernutrition is closely related to household food security — the ability to produce or buy adequate, safe and good quality food to meet the dietary requirements of all family members at all times. While most undernutrition occurs in poor countries, it can also occur among older women in privileged societies, in pockets of poverty, social isolation or neglect. The loss of teeth and a lack of access to dental care exacerbates eating and nutrition problems among older people. Undernutrition can result in decreased muscular strength, lowered resistance to infection, and inadequate body weight for height, which in turn, can lead to reduced bone mass and fractures, reduced autonomy and higher mortality rates. Accumulating evidence also suggests an important relationship between the incidence of age-related cataracts and nutritional status.[83]

Older women are often excluded from development programmes, including credit schemes, help for small businesses, farming, and community development projects. This is unfortunate since studies show that collectives of ageing women can be highly successful in development projects and in repaying loans, and that older women rely upon a diverse range of activities to sustain themselves and their families.[95]

Women are more likely than men to be widowed. Widows invariably experience a reduction in income and are highly vulnerable to poverty.[96, 97] In some countries, inheritance laws still discriminate against women; in others, it is common practice for male relatives to take possession of a widow's property and possessions, even when the laws demand otherwise. Ageing women who divorce may be even more vulnerable to poverty than widows.

Income security benefits and accessible, affordable health services are the bedrock of protecting the well-being of older people. It has been demonstrated that it is feasible to provide older people with a small, universal old-age pension and that whole families benefit from this policy. For example, in Brazil and South Africa, the social pension programmes reach a large number of older people at relatively low cost and attract a large measure of political and public support.[98] Family support and access to health care are also recognized as important pillars to old age security and improved health.[99]

Implications for policy, practice and research

Income and health security. Ultimately each country must decide on the best mix of policies and practices in taxation, income security, health care and social services that are needed to maintain the economic well-being and health of older women.

The most urgent need is to ensure that all older women have access to the basic necessities of life, including food, clean water, shelter, primary health care and social support. Assisting older women who live in poor rural areas and in urban slums will help address some of the world's poorest people.

The second most important need is to increase opportunities for older women to participate in development and anti-poverty programmes, and in productive, paid and decent work when they are able and willing to do so. Providing credit, information, services, training, social security and health care benefits to older women would enhance their productivity and support their efforts to maintain themselves and their families.

Providing a basic old age pension that is not tied to work in the formal sector is one of the best ways to improve older women's health and that of their families. Other policies that will reduce inequities include extending employer-provided pensions and benefits to part-time workers and facilitating access to health security and primary health care through health cooperatives for ageing women who work in the informal sector.

Governments, employers and civil society must ensure that widows and divorced women are not left destitute and excluded by enacting and enforcing laws that prohibit gender discrimination in inheritance practices, access to property, pensions and resources, and cultural practices that harm women whose husbands die or divorce them.

In very old age (80-plus) women far outnumber men in the same age category. It is prudent therefore to encourage women to prepare financially for old age (and in many cases to live alone) and to promote a mix of public and private sources of income in old age. Financial aid and social support should be provided for families who care for older women and men who are unable to live independently.

Support for the caregiving role. By approaching caregiving through a gender lens across the life course, decision-makers, nongovernmental organizations, civil society and the private sector can promote family-friendly solutions that address the disproportionate financial burden that caregiving imposes upon women.[100] Childcare and eldercare require policies that protect caregivers from losing their jobs or receiving reduced benefits, and provide employers with incentives to support the care of dependent family members.

A coordinated response to HIV/AIDS must acknowledge and financially support the caregiving roles and contributions of older people (and particularly grandmothers) in the fight against HIV/AIDS. Enabling the participation and representation of older people, and older women in particular, in HIV/AIDS programme planning at local, district

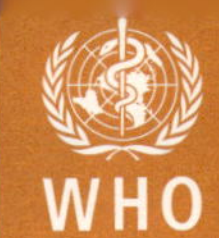

and national levels will help to improve the lives of all who are infected and affected by HIV/AIDS.

Changing attitudes. Many societies view older people and older women in particular as a drain on society. In their efforts to reduce poverty and improve the quality of life for older women, policy-makers and practitioners need to envisage them not only as recipients of protection and assistance, but also as agents of change and development who can help identify solutions for the problems affecting them.

International solidarity. Despite the fact that poverty is usually greater in old age and that gender is a cross-cutting issue in all the Millennium Development Goals, no specific mention is made of older women and men in the prescribed goals, targets and indicators. This exclusion of older people may contribute to the failure to reach the Millennium Development Goals by 2015, unless remedial action is taken. For instance, the non-contributory pension schemes that have been adopted in Brazil and South Africa indicate that households which comprise an older person are less poor than those which do not. The pension received by the older person is often the only regular source of income for the entire family, providing access to credit and resources to buy food, medicine and other essentials for not only the older person but also for his/her family. [98]

Research. A better economic analysis is needed to improve the visibility of work involving in informal care and to assure that this work is included in the national and global picture of social and economic statistics. Other research and information dissemination priorities include identifying:

- effective ways to reduce poverty and increase older women's participation in development activities;

- the long-term impact of informal care-giving in various settings, from both the perspective of the caregiver and the care recipient — especially in relation to HIV/AIDS, dementia and adult children with disabilities;

- the best 'policy and programme mix' to support older women caregivers;

- effective ways to reduce the gender gap in wage earnings and to encourage ageing women to work longer; and

- effective ways to provide income and health security to ageing women who work in the informal sector, or without wages in the home.

Grandmothers looking after their dying children and AIDS orphans

Grandmothers comprise the majority of older caregivers who care for people with HIV/AIDS and orphans with AIDS. Since they have depleted their resources on medicines and burials and because there are few or no younger adults left to help earn an income, most of these families of the 'young and old' face desperate poverty, accompanied by stigma and isolation. It is estimated that there are over 12 million AIDS orphans in Africa and that this number will more than double over the next decade.[101,102] and yet the older caregivers who look after these orphans are rarely recognized or supported in current HIV/AIDS policies and interventions.

8. Social determinants

This chapter deals with some of the most important social influences on active ageing: education and literacy, violence and abuse, ageism and social exclusion, human rights, social support, and leadership and empowerment. Family support and living arrangements are covered in the section on the physical environment.

Key points

People with a low level of education have shorter lives and fewer years in good health than people with a higher level of education. Some studies have shown that this inequality in health expectancy is greater in women than men.[103,104]

Worldwide, women age 60 and over have extraordinarily high levels of illiteracy, and the gender gap between women and men is predicted to persist.[105] Older indigenous women bear the burden of the highest rates of illiteracy, even in countries with high literacy levels. This limits their ability to be active citizens, workers and members of their society, and infringes on their access to fundamental human rights.[106]

Older women are vulnerable to loneliness due to their greater longevity, and incur a high likelihood of being widowed, living alone, and experiencing an increased number of years with declining health.[107] At the same time, women are more likely than men to have a social support network centred on close relationships with family members and friends.[108]

Social exclusion is often the result of discrimination based upon gender, age, race, ethnicity, ability and socioeconomic status. Older, minority women may face triple jeopardy and suffer poor health as a result of social exclusion based on barriers to education, work, citizenship and health care. Older women in transitional societies such as those in eastern and central Europe may experience a deep sense of social isolation, in the face of massive political and social upheaval and unemployment, in addition to the early deaths of their husbands.[109]

Widows are particularly vulnerable to social exclusion. In addition to the reduction in income that invariably follows the death of one's spouse, widows in some cultures suffer social stigma, taboos, and restrictions that are detrimental to their mental and physical health. For example, the approximately 33 million widows in India are expected to lead chaste, isolated and austere lives.[110]

Older women are more likely than older men to engage in volunteer work in the community. In Australia, the value of unpaid voluntary work outside the home by older women is estimated to range from AU$670 to AU$975 per woman per year.[111]

Abuse and gender-based violence in the home and community affects older women.[112] Many older women who are abused or neglected were and sometimes still are caregivers to those who abuse them; parents who provide their adult children and/or grandchildren with food, shelter, spending money and love; or partners who are looking after spouses who have been diagnosed with a chronic illness. In conflict and situations where law has broken down, isolated older women are not excluded in the widespread incidences of rape and other human rights violations linked to gender-based violence.[113]

Older women, like other groups in society, must have legal protection for the full range of internationally accepted human rights. Despite being signatories to the UN Convention on the Elimination of all Forms of Discrimination Against Women (CEDAW), many countries still discriminate against ageing women through unequal rights to marry, divorce, acquire nationality, inherit property, seek employment, be protected from abuse and obtain access to credit and health care.[114]

Older women are under-represented in positions of leadership and power at community, national, and international levels. This is especially true for women in low-income circumstances where the interaction between poverty and social exclusion creates barriers to social, political, and economic participation.

Ageism (negative attitudes and discrimination based on age) is a concern for both women and men; however, it can be particularly problematic for ageing women. The media and prevailing attitudes often portray men as ageing with wisdom, while women become 'invisible' in middle-age and are viewed as a burden in older age. This disadvantage is, in part, due to a tendency to equate women's worth with beauty, youth, and reproduction.

> ### Elder abuse
>
> Elder abuse is "a single or repeated act, or lack of appropriate action, occurring within any relationship where there is an expectation of trust, which causes harm or distress to an older person". Older women who are abused are more likely to suffer from depression, anxiety and physical disabilities. The effects may also be fatal as a result of homicide, severe injury, neglect, or suicide.[112]

Implications for policy, practice and research

Education and literacy. Eliminating gender disparity in primary and secondary education (one of the Millennium Development Goals) will help improve literacy levels in generations to come. At the same time, it is essential to address the literacy needs of ageing cohorts now. Governments, civil society, and employers need to make special efforts to support the participation of midlife and older women in literacy, skills and job training, and lifelong learning activities.

Social support and social exclusion. Policies and practices that encourage social support and discourage social exclusion include those that:

- involve older women in all levels of planning and remove the social barriers to participation;

- increase opportunities for older people – especially those who live alone, are disabled or are members of minority groups – to interact;

- foster intergenerational activities and relationships;

- reach out to widows and members of indigenous populations; and

- encourage and enable older women to make use of their productive potential by volunteering for work.

Elder abuse and societal violence. A comprehensive approach to the prevention and amelioration of violence against women of all ages includes strengthening the capacity of law enforcement and justice officials to respond to complaints. This response should include protecting the victims and punishing the perpetrators, establishing support services in the community and supporting collaborative efforts with nongovernmental organizations. Groups working in the areas of ageing and women's rights need to advocate for these actions on behalf of older – as well as younger – women. Grandfathers, fathers and male leaders can assert the responsibility of men to condemn gender and age stereotyping and to commit to preventing crimes against women of all ages.

Cruel and violent practices against widows and older women who are branded as witches must be stopped. Policy-makers and law enforcement officials need to be aware that violent acts such as rape and slavery in lawless situations affect older – as well as younger – women. Action must be taken to deal with and prevent atrocities committed against older women such as rape and sexual coercion, as well as street crimes and financial abuse.

Ageism and human rights. Policies need to adopt a rights-based approach that allocates older women their fair share of national and global resources, and is faithful to the United Nations Principles for Older People: independence, participation, care, self-fulfilment and dignity.

Parents and teachers, business leaders, nongovernmental organizations and older women themselves all have key roles to play in changing misconceptions and negative attitudes towards ageing women. It is particularly important to encourage the media to make ageing women more visible through increased attention to their contributions, needs and rights.

Leadership and empowerment. Supporting the development of organizations for older people, networks, and self-help and advocacy groups will help empower older women and strengthen their capacity to represent their own interests. Women's groups need to encourage older women to participate and take leadership roles, and to ensure that advocacy and educational efforts for

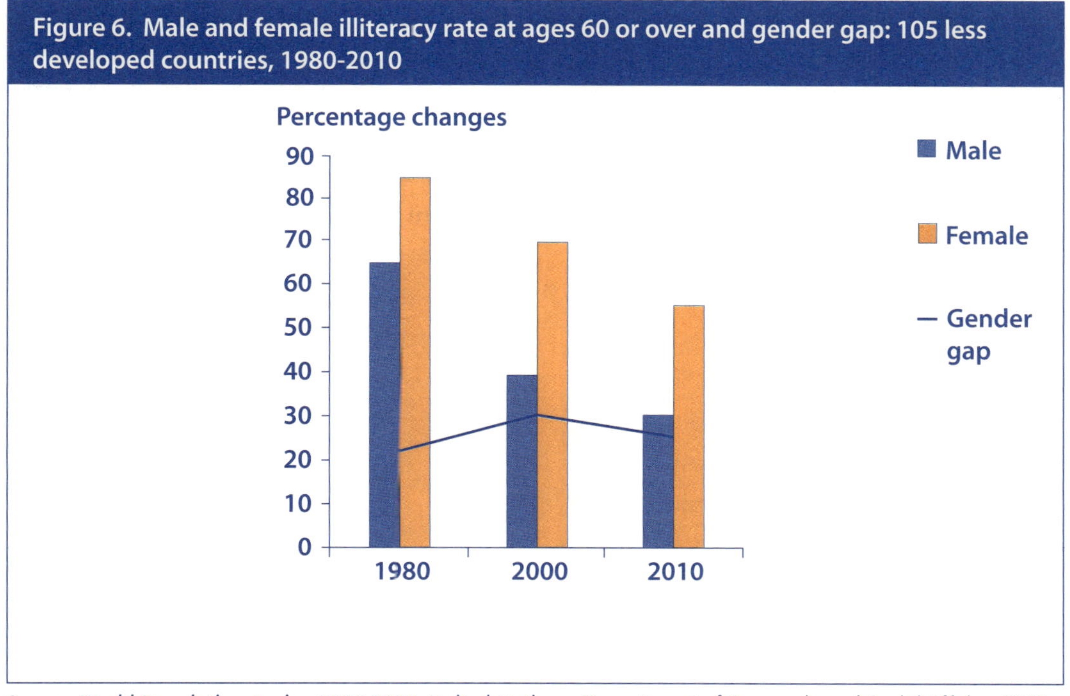

Figure 6. Male and female illiteracy rate at ages 60 or over and gender gap: 105 less developed countries, 1980-2010

Source: World Population Ageing 1950-2050. United Nations, Department of Economic and Social Affairs, 2005

women's health and rights include those of older women. International measures of gender equity should be applied and expanded to document the ages of women leaders in business, politics and academia.

Research and information dissemination. Areas requiring further investigation include:

- how best to address inequities in literacy and education among current cohorts of older women and to ensure that future cohorts have better access to literacy and lifelong learning opportunities;

- how to best address the social exclusion of widows and the infringement on their human rights in some cultures;

- accurate reporting of the levels of elder abuse, domestic violence and community violence experienced by older women and older men;

- best practices to address elder abuse and violence against older women and older men in all its forms;

- the treatment and coverage of older women by the media;

- infringements upon and policies and practices related to the human rights of older women (e.g. rights to inheritance, property, marriage, health care); and

- participation of older women in politics and leadership roles.

9. The physical environment

Key points

Gender, sex and age interact to make older women particularly vulnerable to hazards in the physical environment.

Older women are particularly vulnerable to illness and death related to indoor air pollution. Indoor air pollution that results from burning coal and solid fuels to meet basic energy and cooking needs is a public health tragedy, resulting in nearly 500 000 deaths each year among women.[115]

Extreme weather conditions strongly affect older people. In 2003, when record-high temperatures in Europe claimed an estimated 35,000 lives, most of the victims were older citizens and people with chronic illnesses. In very cold climates, older women are particularly vulnerable to mortality in winter[116] and to broken bones resulting from falls on icy streets and sidewalks.

In developing countries most older women live with family members. In situations of co-residency with family members, there is most often an agreeable exchange of services and support. Older women often supply a significant amount of services (such as child care and domestic duties) that benefit younger people. But rapid social and economic changes combined with a reduced pool of caregivers, have put enormous pressures on families and kin. Some families are unable to share their small homes with older relatives. In some cases, older women who live with their families are neglected, abused or abandoned in the face of unemployment, overcrowded housing, alcohol abuse and gender discrimination exacerbated by age and frailty.

Older women have become increasingly likely to live alone in the last several decades. This trend has been most noticeable in industrialized countries although it is beginning to happen in developing countries as well. Older women who live alone and tend to be divorced or widowed are more likely to experience greater levels of poverty and to be institutionalized than those who live with family members. They are also more likely to feel isolated and depressed, and to require services from the state in the form of home help — although family members (particularly daughters who live nearby) still provide the majority of care and support. [117-119]

In developing countries, when men and young women migrate in search of work, older women often become heads of households. In these situations, distance and access to public transport become primary factors in terms of mutual support. When adult children are unable to travel home regularly, older people ultimately receive reduced social support and the little financial help that children had promised to send home may not arrive.[120]

Ensuring that older women have access to affordable, safe, and appropriate shelter is central to their well-being.[121] Older women who are widowed may find that they cannot afford to repair or modify their house to meet their age-related needs. Those who live in dwellings in poor repair are at especially high risk of falls.

Women and girls in households without electricity or piped water are heavily burdened with the tasks of water and fuel collection. This can lead to musculoskeletal pain and disability in later life. Some 1.7 billion people currently lack access to safe water and this number is expected to reach 2.3 billion by 2025.[122] Surveys in Africa and Asia show that more than half of households in rural areas are without electricity.[123]

Older women are especially vulnerable in disaster situations because they lack information, mobility and resources. Those that survive face desperate circumstances and barriers related to access to shelter and food. At the same time, older women make an important contribution during emergencies (for example, as caregivers and birth attendants). These capacities are seldom acknowledged and older women are rarely included in decision-making and leadership roles related to disaster risk reduction, management and recovery.[124, 125]

Accessible public transportation is critical for maintaining independence, and carrying out everyday tasks such as shopping, getting to appointments and socializing. This is especially important for older women because they usually carry out these duties and even in developed countries they are less likely than men to have access to a car.

The cost of falls

The consequences of falling are more likely to be severe among women because of lower bone density and the higher incidence of osteoporosis. Approximately 2 million hip fractures are estimated to occur worldwide in 2025, the great majority among older women. Hip fracture almost always leads to hospitalization and often causes death. Convalescence is prolonged and many women never return to the same level of functioning.[61] Efforts to prevent falls can mean large savings to the health care system. For example, the Public Health Agency of Canada estimates that a reduction in falls by 20% could result in an estimated 7,500 fewer hospitalizations and approximately $138 million annually could be saved nationally.[126]

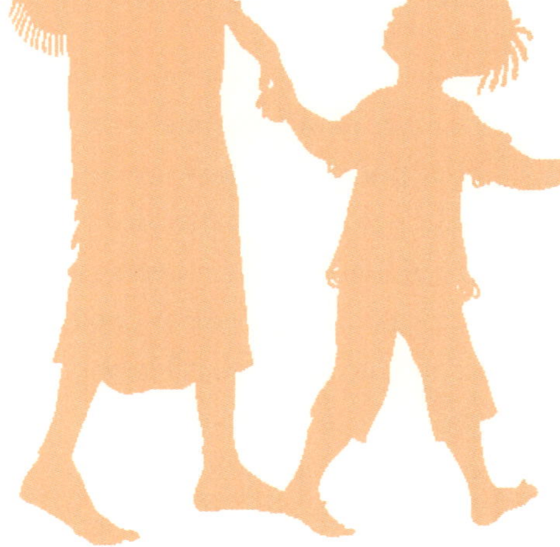

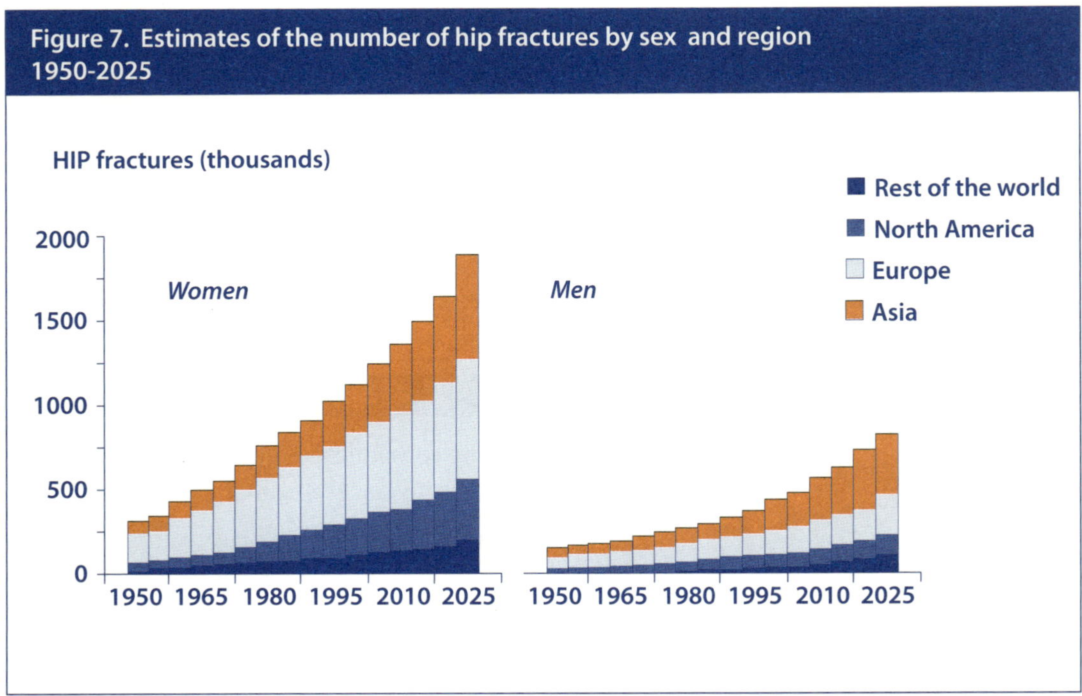

Source: *Prevention and Management of Osteoporosis.* Report of a WHO Scientific Group. World Health Organization, 2003

Implications for policy, practice and research

Indoor air pollution. In the short term, deaths and disability caused by indoor air pollution from solid fuels can be reduced and prevented by better stoves and housing designs. In the longer term, the use of cleaner fuels and electricity can eliminate this public health tragedy.

Housing and living arrangements. As the number of older women who live alone continues to increase around the world, policy-makers need to ensure that a variety of living arrangements are available. In situations where independent living is economically impossible or culturally inappropriate, it is important to foster intergenerational relationships and co-residency by supporting families who care for older relatives, housing designs that enable multi-generational living and community centres that can be used by older people as meeting places and clubs.[127]

Ageing in place adapting to functional impairments without moving from "home" is the choice of most people. Older women may require help with home repairs and other services. The use of new technologies to enable older people to remain independent in their homes has great potential.

Age-friendly cities and communities will address many of the factors in the physical environment that help determine the state of older women's health, such as barrier-free interior and exterior spaces; public spaces that encourage active leisure and socialization; appropriate, accessible housing;

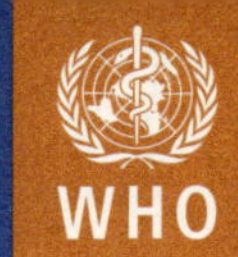

hazard-free streets, sidewalks and buildings; safe, accessible public transportation; and secure, supportive neighbourhoods.

Local governments are uniquely positioned to support age-friendly built environments by coordinating decision-making, promoting awareness and implementing community design plans, strategies and policies that support age-friendly environments.[128]

Disaster and emergencies. When formulating disaster relief and reduction measures, policy-makers and nongovernmental organizations need to systematically assess gender- and age-based vulnerabilities, needs and strengths. This assessment is needed to ensure equal access for women and men of all ages to services at all stages of a relief effort, and to include older women in disaster risk reduction, environmental management and recovery activities. Cash transfers to older people are a vital lifeline in the rebuilding process and will benefit both older people and their families.[125]

Research and information dissemination. Priority areas for increasing our understanding of how to make physical environments more age-friendly and gender-responsive, include:

- innovative and practical ways to make transportation and buildings more accessible for older people with disabilities;

- pros and cons of living arrangement options for older women who live alone;

- how best to support families who provide a home to older women;

- innovative housing options, especially for older women who are poor and alone;

- effective strategies for preventing falls in a variety of settings;

- ways to reduce mortality and morbidity linked to pollution (outdoors and indoors) and extreme weather conditions;

- application of new technologies and designs for assisted living in the community; and

- application and evaluation of age-friendly principles and interventions in urban and rural settings.

The WHO Global Age-friendly Cities project

In 2006 WHO initiated the Global Age-friendly Cities project with partners in several countries. Partners first consult with older persons, and then with community leaders and experts to identify the major physical and social barriers to active ageing. Each partner uses this knowledge to develop, implement and evaluate local action plans to make the environment more age-friendly. To share the findings, WHO compiled the results into practical 'age-friendly city' guidelines that could be used by cities around the world. [129]

10. Moving ahead

This report provides a comprehensive framework for taking action. Decision-makers will need to decide how best to address – within their own settings – the key findings and implications described in this report. This should be done in consultation with ageing women themselves, nongovernmental organizations and civil societies, academics, and professionals working in health care, economics, the labour market, housing, transportation and other sectors. In so doing, it is critical to recognize that improving health requires intersectoral action in a variety of spheres and working collaboratively towards a common goal of improved public health for all.

No single organization, group, or sector is likely to have sufficient resources to tackle the complex issues related to the gendered dimensions of ageing. This is all the more true because the solutions needed to ensure active ageing often fall outside the health sector. Partnerships and collaboration among organizations and sectors is essential.

Nongovernmental organizations concerned with gender, as well as with those concerned with ageing issues, have a key role to play in advocating and enabling policy and practice changes at local, regional, national and international levels. Leaders in these two areas must work together to ensure that both age and gender lenses are simultaneously applied to policy and programme development.

Taking action

Active ageing pillar 1: health and health care

Numerous international agreements affirm the right of all people to the highest possible level of health and access to appropriate health care services. However, older women are often forgotten, ignored or invisible in efforts to achieve health for all — even though they are often crucial to the realization of this goal. Decision-makers can redress these inequities through policies that enable active ageing and address the key issues described in this report. Because of the potential costs associated with living for many years with illness or disability, and the important contributions that ageing women make to informal health care, investing in their health is both a humanitarian and economic necessity.

Priority areas for action include:

- reducing the dramatic inequities in life expectancy among different groups of women both within and among countries and regions;

- establishing or strengthening programmes, policies, services and research efforts that address the prevention and management of chronic diseases and conditions that significantly affect ageing women. Particular attention needs to be paid to disabling conditions such as arthritis, osteoporosis and dementia; eliminating inequalities in vision care

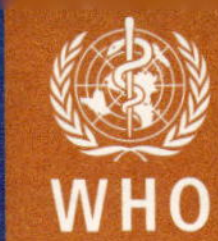

and in the management and treatment of health problems (such as heart disease) that have traditionally been considered 'male' diseases; and introducing new technologies like a vaccine to prevent cervical cancer as well as widely using established technologies e.g. pap smear screening for older women in low and middle-income countries;

- establishing or strengthening programmes, policies, services and research efforts that promote mental health and manage mental illnesses that affect older people. For many women, it is especially important to increase awareness about and reduce the stigma associated with depression; to protect the rights and dignity of older people with Alzheimer disease and other forms of dementia; to reduce gender-based stereotyping related to menopause and the use of psychotropic drugs; and to support the mental health of older people who have experienced elder abuse or other forms of violence at any stage of their lives;

- improving ageing women's access to a continuum of quality care that is both age- and gender-responsive, with an increased emphasis on health promotion for all age groups;

- creating age-friendly, gender-responsive primary health care services;

- providing gender-responsive options in long-term care and palliative care in both community and residential settings;

- informing ageing women about healthy sexuality, HIV/AIDS and other STIs, and providing high-quality services related to reproductive health throughout the life course;

- recognizing and supporting the essential role that grandmothers play as caregivers for people with HIV/AIDS and subsequently as surrogate parents for grandchildren and other AIDS orphans;

- creating environments that enable and encourage girls, young women and older women to be physically active, to refrain from tobacco use, to eat nutritious foods and to maintain a healthy weight. This approach includes the adoption of gender-responsive, comprehensive strategies in tobacco control, physical activity and diet;

- building capacity among health and social service professionals who work with older people by providing training concerning how gender and sex influence health;

- recognizing and supporting the essential contribution that ageing women make as caregivers and major providers of informal health care; and

- reducing gender-related exposure to second-hand smoke and to indoor air pollution from cooking fuels.

Active ageing pillar 2: participation

During the last 20-30 years, the world's governments have affirmed their commitment to promote and protect the full enjoyment of human rights and participation by all women throughout their life course. CEDAW (1979), the International Conference on Population Development (Cairo, 1994), the Fourth World Conference on Women (Beijing, 1995) and the Second World Assembly on Ageing (Madrid, 2002) were central to a major policy shift in this direction. But progress has remained uneven and many challenges remain. One of these challenges is the full inclusion of women in general, and older women in particular, who often face discrimination based on both age and gender in many sectors of society.

Ageing women make substantial economic and social contributions to society. They also represent an important and growing political constituency in both developed and developing countries. Recognizing and supporting their full participation – regardless of socioeconomic status and ethnicity – will benefit the health and well-being of individuals, families, communities and nations.

Priority areas for action include:

- dispelling misconceptions, negative attitudes and stereotypes about older women;

- empowering older women to take an active role in economic growth and the development process;

- improving opportunities for ageing women to engage in decent work when they want to or need to do so. This requires policies that remove employment barriers and age- and gender-based discrimination; recognize work in the informal sector of the economy; and support employers who respond to the needs of ageing women facing intensive long- or short-term caregiving demands;

- supporting intergenerational efforts and cooperation to improve the economic, social and physical well-being of both the older and younger generations;

- recognizing, valuing and supporting the unpaid work that ageing women do in the home and community;

- addressing the literacy needs of ageing women and redressing the large gender gaps in literacy levels between women and men;

- providing equal access to primary, secondary and tertiary education for girls and boys, and to lifelong learning and training opportunities for ageing women and men;

- supporting the social inclusion of all ageing women and reaching out to isolated older women by creating environments that enable their physical and social involvement in community life;

- supporting organizations and groups that are working to develop ageing women's empowerment and leadership capacities at all levels; and

- involving older women in decision-making related to political, social, spiritual and economic issues at all levels.

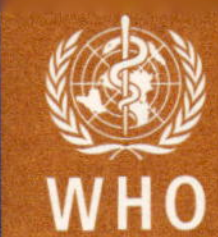

Active ageing pillar 3: security

Poverty and poor health go hand-in-hand. Through the first Millennium Development Goal, governments and international agencies have committed to reducing and eliminating poverty. All over the world women are poorer than men, and in most countries, female poverty deepens with age. Despite this situation, and the fact that gender is a cross-cutting issue in all the Millennium Development Goals, no specific mention is made of older people in the prescribed goals, targets and indicators. Similarly, as awareness and action to confront violence and abuse against younger women gain support within the health sector and beyond, older women consistently remain outside the scope of most advocacy campaigns, direct interventions and research. A lack of policies and programmes that ensure the rights of older women and enhance their economic and physical security jeopardizes their health and their ability to remain active contributors to their families, communities and nations.

Priority areas for action include:

- preventing and reducing poverty among older women, especially older women who live alone and those in indigenous and minority groups who suffer additional discrimination;

- reducing income inequities between various groups of older women both within and among cities, countries and regions;

- providing equitable access to sustainable social security options for older women — including non-contributory pensions;

- providing equal access to health security and health services for older women and men;

- ensuring food security and safe, secure living arrangements for older women;

- preventing, reducing and eliminating elder abuse and violence against ageing women in all its different forms;

- ensuring respect for widows' rights to property, dignity, freedom of movement and self-fulfilment; and

- ensuring that ageing women's human rights are respected and protected — particularly in times of emergency, disaster, and conflict.

Building a research agenda

This report highlights some of the research and knowledge gaps that hamper our ability to formulate policies and programmes that reduce gender inequities and effectively promote active ageing. This section summarizes some key priorities for knowledge development and sharing under each of the three pillars of active ageing. Underlying each of these is the urgent need for increased surveys, studies, and policy analyses in developing countries. Developed countries can play a key role in improving our understanding of the global picture of ageing women's health by providing technical assistance and funding for research efforts in less developed countries.

Health and health care

Increase our understanding of health issues related to ageing in women and the effectiveness of various interventions, through the following measures:

- Include ageing women in all medical research and clinical trials on diseases and health conditions that affect them, both as subjects and in advisory functions.

- Ensure that all data are age- and sex-disaggregated and published in that format, and extend all data gathering to include the oldest old (age 80-plus).

- Priority areas for developing and sharing knowledge should be centred on strengthening primary health care and include:

  - ageing women's experience with abuse and violence, in terms of cumulative exposure and in exposure specific to older age;

  - ageing women's experience with HIV and AIDS;

  - the modern experience of midlife in a variety of cultures and settings, including the physical and sociocultural changes related to menopause;

  - the experience of widowhood in a variety of settings and cultures;

  - how the social determinants of health differentially affect disease causality and health status (both mental and physical) among women and men;

  - the long-term impact of informal caregiving in various settings from both the perspective of the caregiver and the care recipient — especially in relation to HIV/AIDS, dementia and adult children with disabilities;

  - gender perspectives, expectations and experiences of long-term care options; and

  - more detailed evidence on the differential use of medications by older women and men and whether gender is systematically associated with inappropriate use.

Participation

Increase our understanding of issues and solutions related to the participation of older women in work, development, education, training and literacy, community activities, and leadership roles through the following measures:

- Include older women at each stage of the research, and make use of both quantitative and qualitative methods.

- Make use of composite indices such as the Gender Empowerment Measure (GEM) and the Gender Development Index (GDI) which measure women's empowerment at all stages of the life course.

- Clarify the unpaid contribution of ageing women caregivers to the economy and suggest practical ways to recognize and reward this contribution.

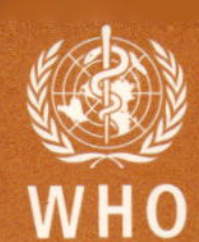

Security

Increase our understanding of security issues and solutions related to gender differences and the experiences of ageing women. Priorities for knowledge development and sharing include:

- elder abuse and violence in the broader community and in times of conflict and disaster;

- the dynamic relationships between living arrangements, intra-family transfers and the health of older people, paying special attention to urban-rural and gender differences; and

- innovative health and social policies that prevent and alleviate poverty among women and their families throughout the life course.

Final Remarks

Policies and practices that support health and active ageing for all will benefit women as well as men. However, it is also critical to understand and act on the gendered dimensions of ageing. Many older women continue to face inequities related to health, security and participation. Often, they face stereotyping and misconceptions that portray them as a burden or as invisible.

On a daily basis and around the world, older women make life better for their peers and succeeding generations, in both small and large ways. It is time to celebrate those contributions and to provide ageing women with full human rights; a positive quality of life, love, and care throughout the life course; and an environment that supports active ageing.

References

1. *Active ageing: a policy framework.* Geneva, World Health Organization, 2002 (available online at: www.who.int/hpr/ageing).

2. *Beijing Declaration and Platform for Action.* Fourth World Conference on Women, Beijing, 1995. New York, United Nations, 1995 (available online at: www.un.org/womenwatch/daw/beijing/platform/index.html).

3. *Madrid International Plan of Action on Ageing.* New York, United Nations, 2002 (available online at: www.un.org/esa/socdev/ageing/4).

4. *Millennium Development Goals.* New York, United Nations, 2000 (available online at: www.un.org/millenniumgoals).

5. *Gender, women and health: incorporating a gender perspective into the mainstream of WHO's policies and programmes. Report by the Secretariat.* WHO Executive Board, 116th Session. Provisional agenda item 4.4. Geneva, World Health Organization, 2005 (EB116/13).

6. *World Health Report 2006. Working together for health.* Statistical Annex. Geneva, World Health Organization, 2006.

7. *Mapping existing research and identifying knowledge gaps concerning the situation of older women in Europe (MERI). Summary of the European synthesis report.* Corciano, Italy, Older Women's Network, Europe, 2005 (available online at: www.own-europe.org).

8. Kalache A, Kickbusch I. A global strategy for healthy ageing. *World health*, 1997, 4:4–5.

9. Aboderin I et al. *Life course perspectives on coronary heart disease, stroke and diabetes: key issues and implications for policy and research.* Geneva, World Health Organization, 2002.

10. Ben-Shlomo Y, Kuh D. A life course approach to chronic disease epidemiology: conceptual models, empirical challenges and interdisciplinary perspectives. *International Journal of Epidemiology*, 2002, 31:285–293.

11. Bartley M, Blane D, Montgomery S. Health and the life course: why safety nets matter. *British Medical Journal*, 1997, 314:1194–1196.

12. Wilkinson R, Marmot M, eds. *The solid facts. Social determinants of health*, 2nd ed. Copenhagen, World Health Organization Office for Europe, 2005 (available online at: www.who.dk/document/e81384.pdf).

13. Centers for Disease Control (CDC). *Deaths: final data for 2002.* Washington, DC, United States National Vital Statistics Reports, 2004:53(5).

14. Des Meules M, Manuel D, Cho R. Mortality, life and health expectancy of Canadian women. *Women's Health Surveillance Report.* Ottawa, Canadian Institute for Health Information and Health Canada, 2003.

15. *The health and welfare of Australia's aboriginal and Torres Strait islander peoples.* Canberra, Australian Bureau of Statistics and Australian Institute of Health and Welfare, 1999 (Catalogue No. 4704.0).

16. *International Decade of the World's Indigenous People. Report by the Secretariat.* Fifty-fourth World Health Assembly. Geneva, World Health Organization, 2001.

17. *Aboriginal peoples of Canada.* Ottawa, Statistics Canada (www.12.statcan.ca/english/census01/Products/Analytic/companion/abor/canada.cfm, accessed 2006).

18. *London divided: income inequities and poverty in the capital.* London, Greater London Authority, 2002 (available online at: www.london.gov.uk).

19. *Preventing chronic diseases: a vital investment.* Geneva, World Health Organization, 2005 (available online at: www.who.int/chp/chronic_disease_report/en).

20. *Gender and blindness. Fact sheet.* Geneva, Department of Gender and Women's Health, World Health Organization, 2002.

21. *Women's mental health: an evidence based review.* Geneva, World Health Organization, 2000 (available online at: www.who.int).

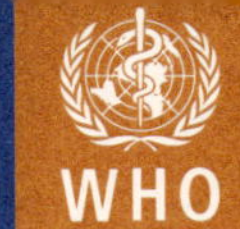

22. Patel V, Kleinman A. Poverty and common mental disorders in developing countries. *Bulletin of the World Health Organization*, 2003, 81:609–615.

23. *World Health Report 2001. Mental health: new understanding, new hope.* Geneva, World Health Organization, 2001 (available online at: www.who.int).

24. Brookmeyer R, Gray S. Methods for projecting the violence and prevalence of chronic diseases in aging populations: application to Alzheimer's disease. *Statistics in Medicine*, 2000, 19(11–12):1481–1493.

25. *Distribution of suicide rates by age and gender*, 2000. Geneva, World Health Organization, 2002 (available online at: www.who.int/mental_health/prevention/suicide).

26. Matthews K, Wing R, Kuller L. Influences of natural menopause on psychological characteristics and symptoms of middle-aged healthy women. *Journal of Consulting and Clinical Psychology*, 1990, 58:345–363.

27. Sorensen S, Pinquart M, Duberstein P. How effective are interventions with caregivers? An updated meta-analysis. *Gerontologist*, 2002, 42(3):356–372.

28. *Prevention of mental disorders, effective interventions and policy options. Summary report.* Geneva, World Health Organization, 2004.

29. *Impact of AIDS on older people in Africa: Zimbabwe case study.* Geneva, World Health Organization, 2002.

30. *The cost of love. older people in the fight against AIDS in Tanzania.* London, HelpAge International, 2004.

31. Leeder S et al. *Race against time: the challenge of cardiovascular disease in developing countries*. New York, Centre for Global Health and Economic Development, 2004.

32. Bath P, Gray L. Association between hormone replacement therapy and subsequent stroke: a meta-analysis. *British Medical Journal*, 2005, 10:1136.

33. National Institutes of Health, National Heart, Lung, and Blood Institute. Results of Women's Health Study. *Journal of the American Medical Association*, 2002, 28(3).

34. Mikhail G. Coronary heart disease is under-diagnosed and under-treated in women [editorial]. *British Medical Journal*, 2005, 331:467.

35. *Preventing cervical cancer worldwide.* Population Reference Bureau and the Alliance for Cervical Cancer Prevention (ACCP), 2005 (available at: www.alliance-cxca.org).

36. Melton L et al. Prevalence and incidence of vertebral deformities. *Osteoporosis International*, 1993, 3:113–119.

37. Li F et al. Enhancing the psychological well-being of elderly individuals through Tai Chi exercise: a latent growth curve analysis. *Structural Equation Modelling*, 2001, 8(1):53–83.

38. Stevens N, Van Tilburg T. Stimulating friendships in later life: a strategy for reducing loneliness among older women. *Educational Gerontology*, 2000, 26(1):15–35.

39. Mulrow C et al. Quality of life changes and hearing impairment. A randomized trial. *Annals of Internal Medicine*, 1990, 113(3):188–194.

40. Shapiro A, Taylor M. Effects of a community-based early intervention program on the subjective well-being, institutionalization and mortality of low-income elders. *Gerontologist*, 2002, 42(3):334–341.

41. *Prevention and control of influenza pandemics and annual epidemics.* WHO Executive Board, 111th Session. EB111.R6. Agenda item 5.8. Geneva, World Health Organization, 2003 (EB111.R6) (available online at: wholibdoc.who.int/eb/2003/EB111_R6.pdf).

42. Mahalingam K. *Evaluation of cataract surgical service delivery to the visually impaired of Chamrajnagar district, Karnataka State, India.* Copenhagen, Institute of Public Health, University of Copenhagen (pubhealth.ku.dk/mih_en/thesesAbstr/03/mahalingam, accessed 2005).

43. Melese M et al. Indirect costs associated with accessing eye care services as a barrier to service use in Ethiopia. *Tropical Medicine & International Health*, 2004, 9(3):426–431.

44. Britton A et al. Does access to cardiac investigation and treatment contribute to social and ethnic differences in coronary heart disease? Whitehall II prospective cohort study. *British Medical Journal*, 2004, 329(7461):318.

45. Raine R. Does gender bias exist in the use of specialist health care? *Journal of Health Services Research Policy*, 2000, 5:237–249.

46. Hippisley-Cox J et al. Sex inequalities in ischaemic heart disease in general practice: cross sectional survey. *British Medical Journal*, 2001, 322:832.

47. *Older women's health issues paper*. Kanata, ON, Canadian Association on Gerontology, 1998 (available online at: www.cagacg.ca).

48. *Beyond 50: a report to the nation on trends in health security*. Washington, DC, American Association of Retired Persons, 2002.

49. Harwood R, Aihie Sayer A, Hirschfeld M. *Current and future long-term care needs.* An analysis based on the 1990 WHO study The Global Burden of Disease and the International Classification of Functioning, Disability and Health. Geneva, World Health Organization, 2002.

50. *What evidence is there about the effects of health care reforms on gender equity, particularly in health?* Copenhagen, World Health Organization Regional Office for Europe Health Evidence Network, 2005 (available online at: www.euro.who.int/HEN).

51. Whitehead M, Dalgren G, Gilson L. Developing the policy response to inequities in health: a global perspective. In: Evans T et al., eds. *Challenging inequities in health: from ethics to action.* New York, Oxford University press, 2001:35–44.

52. Breen N. Social discrimination and health: gender, race and class in the United States. In: Sen G, George A, Ostlin P, eds. *Engendering international health: the challenge of equity.* Cambridge, MA, MIT Press, 2002.

53. Apt N. Rapid urbanization and living arrangements of older persons in Africa. In: United Nations, Population Division. Living arrangements of older persons: critical issues and policy responses. *Population Bulletin of the United Nations*, 2001, Special Issues 42 and 43:288–310.

54. Resnikoff S et al. Global data on visual impairment in the year 2002. *Bulletin of the World Health Organization*, 2004, 82(11):844–851.

55. *Men, ageing and health: achieving health across the life span.* Geneva, World Health Organization, 2002 (available online at: www.who.int).

56. *Women, ageing and health. Fact sheet.* Geneva, World Health Organization, 2000 (available online at: www.who.int/entity/mediacentre/factsheets/fs252/en).

57. Des Meules M, Turner L, Cho R. Morbidity experiences and disability among Canadian women. In: *Women's Health Surveillance Report.* Ottawa, Canadian Institute Health Information and Health Canada, 2003.

58. Guralnik J et al. Health and social characteristics of older women with disability. *The Women's Health and Aging Study.* Washington, National Institute on Aging, 2000.

59. Genant H et al. Interim report and recommendations of the World Health Organization Task-Force for Osteoporosis. *Osteoporosis International.* 1999, 10(4):259–264.

60. Roubenoff R, Hughes V. Sarcopenia: current concepts. *Journals of Gerontology Series A: Biological Sciences and Medical Sciences*, 2000, 55(12):M716–724.

61. WHO Scientific Group. *Prevention and management of osteoporosis.* Geneva, World Health Organization, 2003 (WHO Technical Report Series, No. 921).

62. Guthrie J et al. The menopausal transition: a 9-year prospective population-based study. The Melbourne Women's Midlife Health Project. *Climacteric*, 2004, 7:375–389.

63. North American Menopause Society. Recommendations for estrogen and progestogen use in peri- and postmenopausal women: October 2004 position statement. *Menopause: The Journal of The North American Menopause Society*, 2004, 11(6):589–600 (available online at: www.menopause.org).

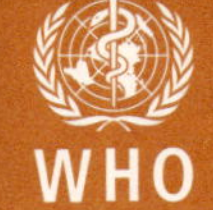

64. *Statement for health professionals.* Australasian Menopause Society, 2004 (available online at: www.menopause.org.au).

65. Barker D, ed. *Fetal and infant origins of adult disease.* London, BMJ Books, 1992.

66. Jetté A, Branch L. The Framingham disability study. II. Physical disability among the aging. *American Journal of Public Health*, 1981, 71(11):1211–1216.

67. Baltes P, Baltes M. *Successful aging: perspectives from the behavioural sciences.* New York, Cambridge University Press, 1990.

68. *Age, gender and HIV/AIDS.* London, HelpAge International, 2002 (HelpAge International Gender and Ageing Briefs) (available online at: www.helpage.org).

69. Wong P. Spirituality, meaning and successful aging. In: Wong PT, Fry P, eds. *The human quest for meaning.* Mahwah, NJ, Lawrence Erlbaum Associates, 1998.

70. Mollard W. Aging and the meaning of life. *Expression*, 1995, 8(4) (available online at: http://64.26.138.100/naca_main).

71. *Gender, health and tobacco.* Fact sheet. Geneva, World Health Organization, 2003 (available online at: www.who.int/gender/documents/en/Gender_Tobacco_2.pdf).

72. *The World Health Report 2002. Reducing risks, promoting healthy life.* Geneva, World Health Organization, 2002.

73. British Medical Association. *Smoking and reproductive life: the impact of smoking on sexual, reproductive and child health.* London/Edinburgh, British Medical Association, Board of Science and Education/Tobacco Control Resource Centre, 2004.

74. Kreuzer M et al. Risk factors for lung cancer among non-smoking women. *International Journal of Cancer*, 2002, 100:706–713.

75. Granville C et al. Mutation spectra of smoky coal combustion emissions in Salmonella reflect the TP53 and KRAS mutations in lung tumors from smoky coal-exposed individuals. *Mutation Research*, 2003, 525:77–83.

76. Keohavong P et al. K-ras mutations in lung carcinomas from non-smoking women exposed to unvented coal smoke in China. *Lung Cancer*, 2003, 41:21–27.

77. Kleinerman R et al. Lung cancer and indoor exposure to coal and biomass in rural China. *Journal of Occupational and Environmental Health*, 2002, 44:338–344.

78. *Growing older, staying well. Ageing and physical activity in everyday life.* Geneva, World Health Organization, 1998 (available online at: www.who.int).

79. *Physical activity for active aging.* Washington, DC, Pan American Health Organization, 2002.

80. O'Brien Cousins S. Promoting active living and healthy eating among older Canadians. *Canadian health action: building on the legacy. Determinants of health – adults and seniors.* Ottawa, National Forum on Health, 1998.

81. Campbell L, Samarask K. Nutrition and physical activity needs of women aged 40 and over. *Medical Journal of Australia*, 2000, 173(Suppl. 6).

82. *Diet, nutrition and the prevention of chronic diseases.* Geneva, World Health Organization, 2003 (WHO Technical Report Series, No. 916).

83. World Health Organization/Tufts University. *Keep fit for life. Meeting the nutritional needs of older persons.* Geneva/Boston, World Health Organization/Tufts University School of Nutrition Science and Policy, 2002.

84. Venning G. Recent developments in vitamin D deficiency and muscle weakness among elderly people. *British Medical Journal*, 2005, 330:524–526.

85. *The state of aging and health in Latin America and the Caribbean.* [Note: data from the Survey on health, well-being and aging in Latin America and the Caribbean (SABE), 1999–2000]. Washington, DC, Pan American Health Organization, 2004.

86. *Global strategy on diet and physical activity. Facts related to chronic diseases.* Geneva, World Health organization, 2005 (available online at: www.who.int/hpr/gs.fs.cvds.shtm).

87. *Diabetes mellitus. Fact sheet 138.* Geneva, World Health Organization, 2002 (available online at: www.who.int).

88. Kelly C, Booth G. Diabetes in Canadian Women. In: *Women's Health Surveillance Report*. Ottawa, Canadian Institute for Health Information, 2003.

89. Booth et al. Diabetes and cardiac disease. In: *Diabetes in Ontario: ICES atlas*. Toronto, Institute for Clinical Evaluative Sciences, 2002.

90. *Framework Convention on Tobacco Control*. Geneva, World Health Organization, 2003 (available online at: www.who.int/tobacco/framework).

91. Mestheneos E, Triantafillou J. *Services for supporting family carers of elderly people in Europe: characteristics, coverage and usage.* Hamburg, Eurofamcare, 2005.

92. *The world's women 2000: trends and statistics.* New York, United Nations, 2000 (available online at: http://unstats.un.org/unsd/demographic/products/indwm/wwpub.htm).

93. *Facts on women at work*. Geneva, International Labour Organization, 2004 (available online at: www.ilo.org/gender).

94. Reday-Mulvey G. Women and the fourth pillar. The four pillars. *Geneva Association Information Newsletter*, 2004, 35 (available online at: www.genevaassociation.org).

95. HelpAge International. *The ageing and development report. Poverty, independence and the world's older people.* London, Earthscan Publications, 1999.

96. Giri V, Khanna M. *Status of widows of Vrindavan and Varanasi: a comparative study.* New Delhi, Guild of Service, 2002 (available online at: http://griefandrenewal.com/widows_study.htm).

97. Munnell A. *Why are so many older women poor? Just the facts on retirement.* Chestnut Hill, MA, Centre for Retirement Research at Boston College, 2004 (available online at: http://www.bc.edu/cit).

98. *Non-contributory pensions and poverty prevention. A comparative study of Brazil and South Africa,* London, HelpAge International, 2003.

99. Holzmann R et al. *Old-age income support in the twenty-first century: an international perspective on pension systems and reform.* Washington, DC, World Bank, 2005.

100. Weitz T, Estes C. Adding aging and gender to the women's health agenda. *Journal of Women & Aging*, 2001, 3(2):3–20.

101. *Africa's AIDS orphans.* New York, United Nations Children's Fund, 2003.

102. *AIDS epidemic update.* Geneva, UNAIDS, 2001/2004 (available online at: www.unaids.org).

103. Manor O et al. Educational differentials in mortality from cardiovascular disease among men and women: The Israel Longitudinal Mortality Study. *Annals of Epidemiology*, 2004, 14(7):453–460.

104. Bossuyt N et al. Socio-economic inequalities in health expectancy in Belgium. *Public Health*, 2003, 118(1).

105. *World population ageing*, 1950–2050. New York, United Nations Department of Economic and Social Affairs, Population Division, 2005.

106. Reyes Gomez L. Vejez y pobreza: el caso de los zoques de Chiapas.VI Meeting of the Mexican Society of Demography, Mexico City. In: HelpAge International. *State of world's older people.* London, HelpAge International, 2002.

107. Hall M, Havens B. *The effect of social isolation and loneliness on the health of older women.* Winnipeg, Prairie Women's Health Centre of Excellence (www.pwhce.ca/effectSocialIsolation.htm, accessed 2005).

108. Weber M. *She stands alone: a review of the recent literature on women and social support.* Winnipeg, Prairie Women's Health Centre of Excellence, 1998 (available online at: www.pwhce.ca).

109. *A generation in transition: older people's situation and civil society's response in east and central Europe.* London, HelpAge International, 2002 (available online at: www.helpage.org/publications).

110. Alter Chen M. *Perpetual mourning: widowhood in rural India.* Oxford, Oxford University Press, 2000.

111. de Vaus D, Gray M, Stanton S. The value of unpaid work of older Australians. *Family Matters*, 2002, 66:34–39 (Australian Institute of Family Studies).

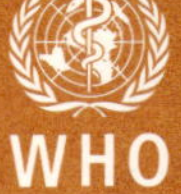

112. *Abuse of the elderly. Fact sheet.* Geneva, World Health Organization, 2002 (available online at: www.who.int/violence_injury_prevention).

113. *Violence and older people: the gendered dimension.* London, HelpAge International, 2002 (HelpAge International Gender and Ageing Briefs) (available online at: www.helpage.org).

114. *Gender equality: striving for justice in an unequal world.* Geneva, United Nations Research Institute for Social Development, 2005.

115. Rehfuess E, Corvalon C, Neira M. Indoor air pollution: 4000 deaths a day must no longer be ignored. *Bulletin of the World Health Organization*, 2006, 84(7):508.

116. Wilkinson P et al. Vulnerability to winter mortality in elderly people in Britain: population based study. *British Medical Journal*, 2004, 329:647.

117. Grundy E. Living arrangements and the health of older people in developed countries. In: United Nations, Population Division. Living arrangements of older persons: critical issues and policy responses. *Population Bulletin of the United Nations*, 2001, Special Issues 42 and 43:311–329.

118. Breeze E, Sloggett A, Fletcher A. Socioeconomic and demographic predictors of mortality and institutional residence among middle aged and older people: results from the Longitudinal Study. *Journal of Epidemiological Community Health*, 1999, 53:765–774.

119. Pendry E, Barrett G, Victor C. Changes in household composition among the over sixties: a longitudinal analysis of the Health and Lifestyles Surveys. *Health and Social Care in the Community*, 1999, 7:109–119.

120. Apt N. Rapid urbanization and living arrangements of older persons in Africa. In: United Nations, Population Division. Living arrangements of older persons: critical issues and policy responses. *Population Bulletin of the United Nations*, 2001, Special Issues 42 and 43:288–310.

121. Thomson H, Petticrew M, Morrison D. *Housing improvement and health gain: a systematic review.* London, Medical Research Council Social and Public Health Sciences, 2001 (Unit Occasional Paper 52) (available online at: http://www.msoc-mrc.gla.ac.uk).

122. *World day for water. News release.* Nairobi/Tokyo, United Nations Environment Programme/United Nations University, 2001 (available online at: www.unesco.org/water/water).

123. United Nations Statistics Division, 2000.

124. *Environmental management and the mitigation of natural disasters: a gender perspective.* New York, United Nations, Division for the Advancement of Women, 2001 (available online at: www.un.org/womenwatch/daw).

125. *Tsunami: the impact on older women and men. Fact Sheet.* London, HelpAge International, 2005 (available online at: www.helpage.org).

126. Public Health Agency of Canada. *Report on seniors' falls in Canada.* Ottawa, Division of Aging and Seniors, Minister of Public Works and Government Services, 2005.

127. *Situations and voices. The older poor and excluded in South Africa and India.* New York, United Nations Population Fund, 2002 (Population and Development Strategies Series, No. 2.

128. *Age-friendly built environments: opportunities for local government.* Perth, Australian Local Government Association, 2004.

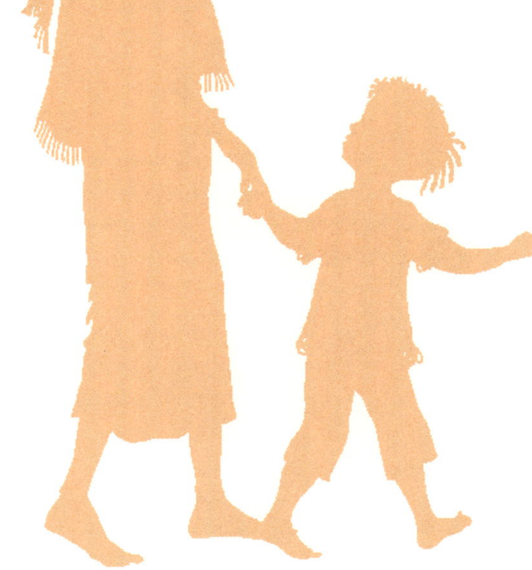